Fresh Face

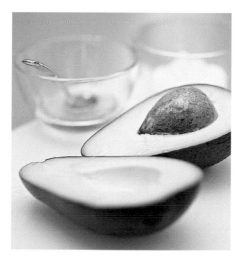

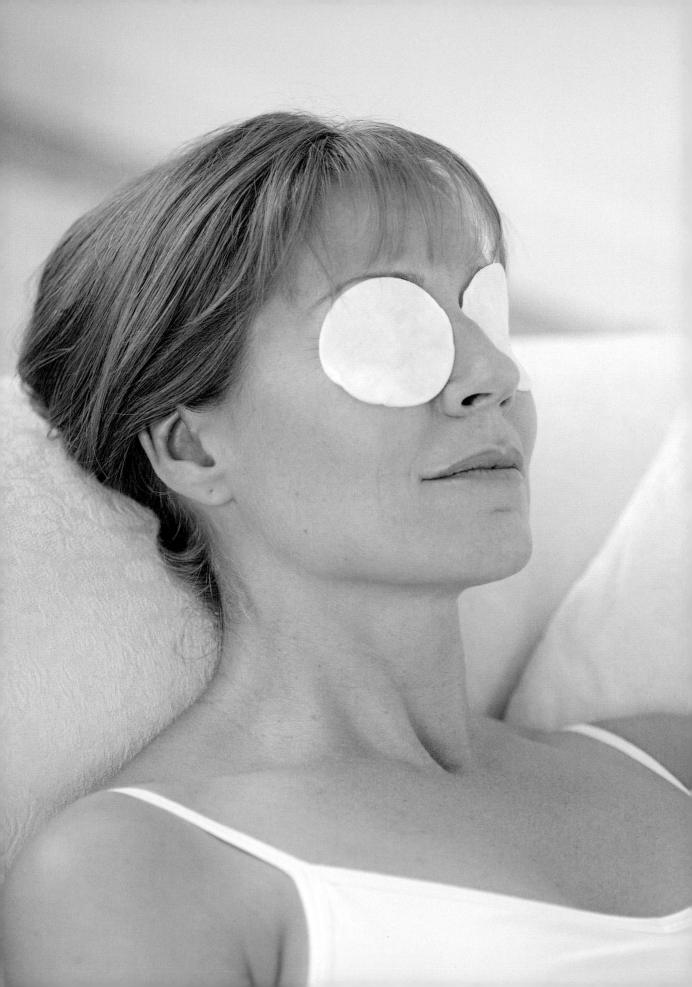

hamlyn

Fresh Face

the easy way to look 10 years younger

Diana Moran

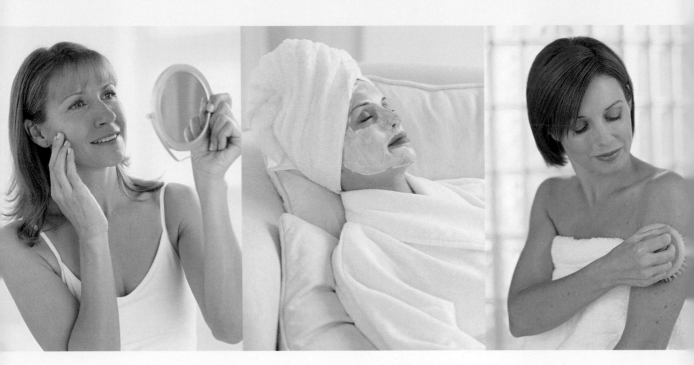

First published in Great Britain in 2005 by
Hamlyn, a division of Octopus Publishing Group Ltd
2–4 Heron Quays, London E14 4JP

Distributed in the United States and Canada by
Sterling Publishing Co., Inc.
387 Park Avenue South, New York, NY 10016-8810

ISBN 0600 61211 2
EAN 9780600612117

A CIP catalogue record for this book is available from the British Library

Printed and bound in China

10 9 8 7 6 5 4 3 2 1

Publisher's note: Massage and facial exercise should not be considered
as a replacement for professional medical treatment; a physician should
be consulted in all matters relating to health. Care should be taken
during pregnancy, particularly in the use of essential oils and pressure
points. Essential oils should not be ingested and should be used for
babies and children only on professional advice.

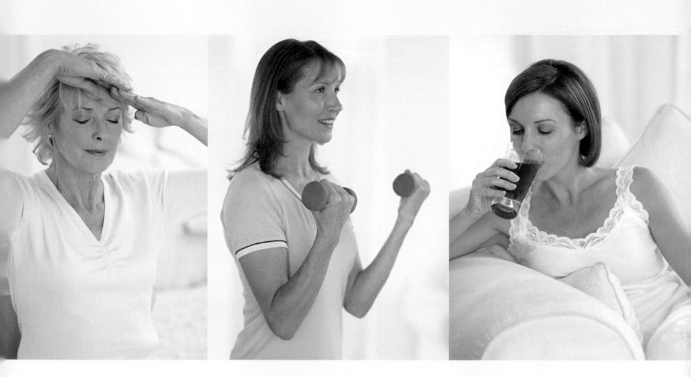

CONTENTS

INTRODUCTION

We can't beat Old Father Time; no – but some women drive a mighty close bargain with him. My career in exercise and wellbeing spans over 40 years, including time spent travelling the world as a fashion and photographic model. I look after my skin and keep in shape – both of which are prerequisites for media success. In 1980, aged 40, I was selected for Oil of Olay's UK and Pan-European TV advertising campaign. I was amazed to be selected again in 1995, aged 55, to launch Oil of Olay's skin care range for mature women. I became the company's worldwide 'face' for extensive media and TV advertising. What a refreshing change – a company using a real live 50-something woman.

Some people think women of 50 are 'past it', but being over 50 myself I enjoy life, am happy with my lifestyle and content with my appearance. I'm not conceited, but dislike media pressure to look 20 years younger. Looking good is about making the most of yourself whatever your age. When we look good, we feel better. People looking after themselves usually glow with good health and lead busy lives.

The facial image a woman presents to the world is not only how she sees herself but also how she wants to be seen by others. Women soon learn tricks to improve upon

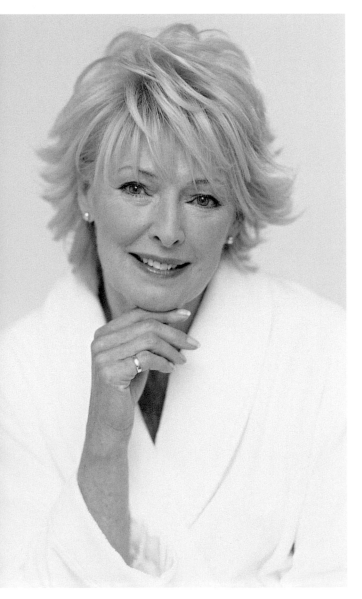

Diana Moran regularly conducts masterclasses in facelifting exercises and is living proof of their effectiveness.

nature, experimenting from an early age with make-up and hairstyles, and finally discovering and developing their own individual style. Women literally 'put on their face' to brave the world. But some women find this process difficult, confused by the variety of beauty products and intimidated by the superior air of some beauty consultants. Some older women become depressed, feeling information and advice dished out by magazines is aimed at 'youngsters' and that they've got nothing left to give or get. Others find that their confidence wanes as the years go by, they stop trying new products or ideas, play safe with old beauty favourites and are too nervous to make changes.

It takes time and money to face the world. When it comes to skin care and beauty products, making mistakes can prove to be very expensive. We might assume that after years of practice, mature women wouldn't make elementary mistakes. But apparently this is not the case, as women's magazines have seen an increase in requests for makeovers and advice from women over 50. Many mature women regard it as frivolous to spend money on themselves. As a result of divorce or bereavement, many women who are over 40 find themselves returning to work, while others suddenly become the main breadwinner, when a husband or partner is made redundant. These newly independent women look for ideas and advice to update their image, but often find themselves having

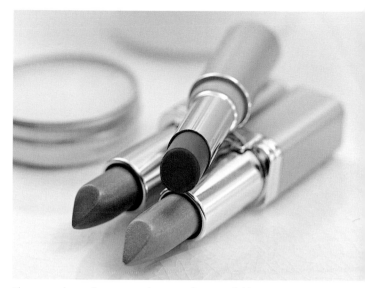

There are plenty of exciting make-up products available to help you achieve a flattering look.

to compete with youngsters of around 18 years of age, both in the workplace and in their social world.

Throughout this book, I share with you tips gleaned from many years in the 'face' business, which I hope will make all mature women feel more confident. Most of us are interested in the latest thinking, advances and techniques in the skin care and beauty business. But to benefit from these, you need to be honest when you look in the mirror and realize that your life and look is constantly changing. Be objective when you face your reflection and learn to appreciate your good points. Only then can you concentrate on, update and improve areas that, with the passing of time, now need a little extra help. So, enjoy. Read the book, learn all the tricks of the trade and, importantly, be comfortable in your own skin.

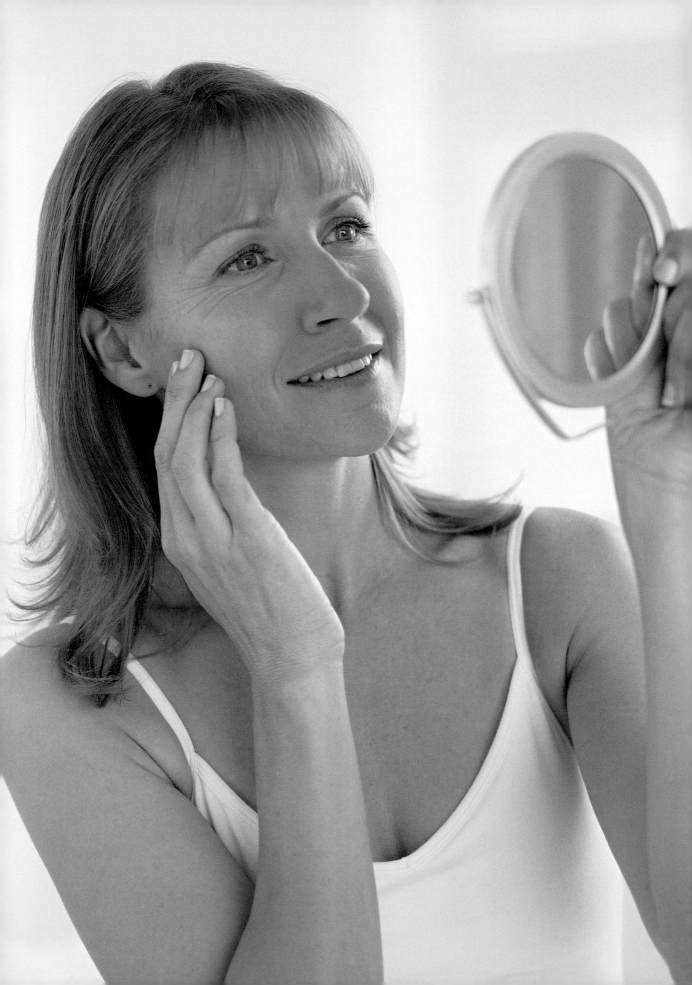

Skin and the ageing process

We cannot turn back the clock, and nor should we want to, but we can learn simple ways to make the most of what we have. Let's start with our bare skin – our base or canvas – on which we can learn to enhance features, disguise faults and create illusions with colour and contour. It is not conceited to take pride in our appearance. When we feel good about ourselves, we are more confident and outgoing, and able to enjoy life to the full. Skin responds to extra care, so let's see how skin ages and then how we can look after it for great, lifelong results.

WHAT IS SKIN?

Skin is the body's only external organ, protecting what is inside and keeping harmful things on the outside. It effectively retains essential fluids, protects internal organs, resists infections and acts as a physical barrier to damage.

Skin plays a vital role in the regulation of our body temperature. In cold climates, the blood vessels in the skin constrict and shrink away from the skin's surface to conserve heat. In hot climates, the skin is flushed, due to blood capillaries moving near the surface in order to lose heat, and is covered with sweat, which evaporates to keep us cool.

Layer upon layer

The skin is not a single layer but has multiple layers containing a complex network of blood vessels and lymph vessels, which deliver nutrients and oxygen, as well as receptors (for pressure, pain and temperature) that send messages to the brain, allowing us to sense our environment.

Skin is responsive and adaptive, with the ability to transform itself according to age, environment, mood, and hormonal and seasonal conditions. A large proportion of the 70 per cent water content of our bodies is found in the skin. Lower layers of the skin contain sensitive nerve receptors, hair follicles that facilitate the movement of lubricating sebum (oil) to the skin's surface and elastic tissues that are able to expand by up to 50 per cent. The uppermost layers display the newly made skin cells and give us our natural complexion. Our bodies constantly make new skin cells: every day millions are produced for facial skin alone.

Is beauty skin deep?

We spend time and money worrying about the thin top layer of the skin, known as the epidermis. Both its colour and its texture matter to us, which is not surprising since we look at it every day. The stratum corneum, the outermost layer of the epidermis, comprises tough, scaly cells that are stuck together with a fatty compound providing skin with its natural protection. These cells are not fresh and new but older cells coming to the end of their days.

New cells are continuously formed in the basal layer – the layer between the epidermis (top) and the dermis (middle); the hypodermis or subcutaneous layer forms the bottom layer. Basal cells are plump and moist as they begin their upward journey to the surface, but change visibly en route. In these cells, the nucleus breaks down and the cells fill with a tough

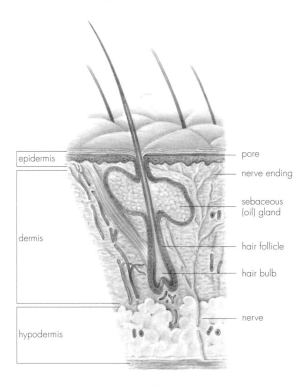

epidermis

dermis

hypodermis

pore

nerve ending

sebaceous (oil) gland

hair follicle

hair bulb

nerve

Each skin cell starts as a moist basal cell, created between the dermis and epidermis.

protein called keratin, becoming drier and flat in the process. Approximately 30 days later they appear on the surface as dead cells, where they are shed naturally. This constant renewal process takes ever-longer as we grow older, and cell turnover decreases with age. But some cells are destroyed prematurely by overexposure to the sun, harmful scavengers (free radicals, see page 14), pollutants, harsh detergents, cleansers and beauty products made from undesirable and avoidable ingredients.

The dermis measures around 3 mm ($\frac{1}{8}$ in) thick and contains hair follicles, nerve endings, blood vessels, connective tissue, sebaceous and sweat glands and collagen fibres, giving skin its youthful appearance, bounce and vitality. Like scaffolding, collagen supports and shapes the skin, while holding everything together. Sadly, the amount of collagen decreases with age, and it is this depletion as we grow older that keeps manufacturers of mature skin-care products in business.

The hypodermis – the lowest layer – is firm, spongy, subcutaneous tissue, containing fat cells, blood vessels, muscles and nerve fibres, all of which are vital for healthy skin.

Face up to ageing

The skin on the face contains more sebaceous glands and nerve endings than other body parts, plus it is supplied with oxygen and nutrients via tiny blood capillaries. It is the finest skin, yet, surprisingly, it is left mostly uncovered and exposed to the elements.

Facial skin is directly attached to over 50 flexible, facial muscles. This tied-in anatomy means that the skin moves with all kinds of expressions, and, as we

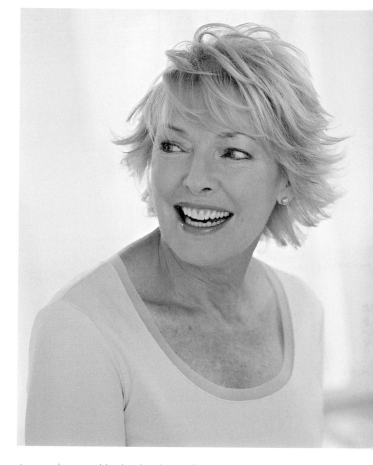

As your skin gets older, laughter lines will set around your mouth; but keep smiling – they're better than frown lines.

get older, these repeated facial expressions start to push the fat in the subcutis into trenches, which, increasingly deprived of their bounce, remain etched on our faces as frown or laughter lines. The faint wrinkles that began in early adult life also deepen, particularly on and around the eyelids and lips.

Over the years, skin loses its pigment, oil production diminishes and less oxygen is carried to the skin's surface. As a result it becomes rougher, its youthful glow fades and the tiredness that can accompany ageing makes the face look older. Even in these enlightened times, far too many women still have a preconception of ageing that causes them to 'act their age'. With this mental attitude, age shows prematurely, but just learning to forget numbers can make women look years younger.

Most unfairly, men tend to retain a more youthful look with age. This is mainly due to male skin being thicker and held in place by facial follicles.

SKIN FACTS

1 sq cm ($\frac{1}{8}$ sq in) of skin contains:

- 2.5 m (8 ft) of nerves
- 1 m (3 ft) of blood vessels
- 3 million cells
- 100 sweat glands
- 12 sebaceous (oil) glands
- 10 hairs

WHAT'S MY SKIN TYPE?

Discover which of the five basic skin types your skin belongs to before considering which products and treatments to buy to keep it in good shape. How well your skin ages depends more on skin type and genetics than on actual age alone.

The five basic skin types are:

- Normal
- Dry
- Oily
- Combination
- Sensitive

Normal skin

This skin type is simply healthy: fresh, smooth and even, neither too oily nor too dry, and with no visible problems. It stays looking good all day and has no reaction to soap and water. If you belong to this rare group, then lucky you. But don't be lulled into a false sense of security: normal skin is still vulnerable to ageing, so always cleanse your skin at night to remove make-up and dirt, and moisturize regularly using a lotion suitable for this skin type.

Dry skin

If you have dry skin, it will be thin, rather translucent in appearance, and liable to chap and flake. Dry skin produces low levels of sebum (the skin's natural moisturizer) and is noticeably flaky around the mouth, cheeks and forehead. Using soap, water and toner causes problems for this skin type, because they leave your skin feeling tight and uncomfortable. When dry skin is exposed to cold winds, central heating or air conditioning, it soon becomes taut. When choosing skin-care products for dry skin, opt for a creamy cleanser, followed by a mild alcohol-free toner to avoid drying out still further. This skin type needs regular feeding with thick, creamy, hydrating moisturizers – morning and night – to keep it in good condition and to avoid the premature ageing to which dry skin is prone.

Oily skin

This skin type is shiny because it produces excessive sebum, especially in the 'T-zone' – the central area of the forehead, nose and chin. Oily skin can have large pores, troublesome blackheads and acne, but it does not react badly to, and is comfortable after, washing with soap and water. Too much soap and water does, however, cause the oil glands to overcompensate and overproduce to combat dryness. The best skin-care routine uses lukewarm water with a facial wash, which is massaged well into the skin and then rinsed off. Avoid alcohol-based astringents, which are too harsh and drying even for oily skins. Use a light moisturizer, the best being a fluid or gel rather than a cream. Wait a few minutes after applying moisturizer and then blot off any that is unabsorbed with a tissue. During the day, refresh the skin by removing excess grease and grime with cotton wool balls soaked in a mild toner.

Combination skin

This mixture of skin types is incredibly common. It combines an oily, large-pored, smooth central skin area (forehead, nose and chin) with an outer, finer-skinned cheek area, which may have rough, dry patches. Each area requires a different skin-care approach. In the morning, treat the T-zone as oily skin: use a facial wash to cleanse and then rinse your whole face. Follow with an alcohol-free toner used only on the T-zone and a mild freshener on drier areas. Keep your skin in tip-top condition by cleansing your entire face with a cream cleanser at night. Use this to remove excess grime with cotton wool balls, followed by a moisturizer applied all over. After 5–10 minutes, remove any excess moisturizer from the oily T-zone with a tissue.

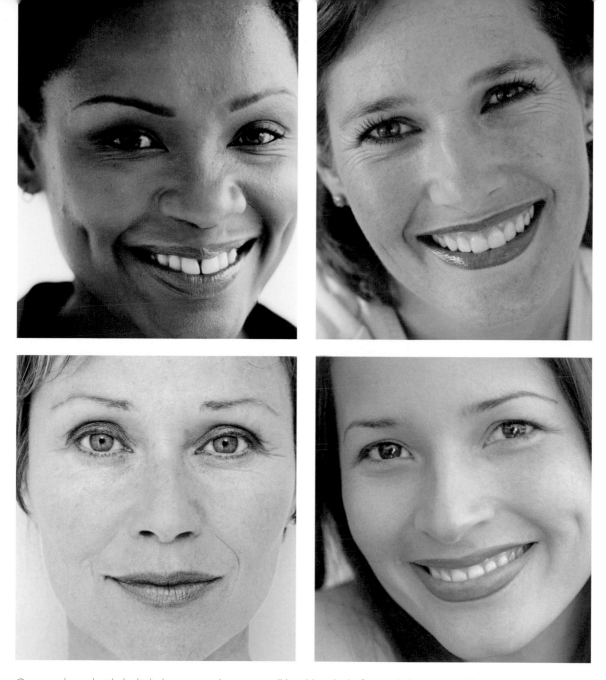

Once you have decided which skin type you have, you will be able to look after it with the most suitable treatments and products.

Sensitive skin

This skin is delicate and difficult to look after. It is usually easily irritated, and reacts to adverse weather conditions, changes in temperatures, sunshine, perfumed products, and harsh ingredients such as detergents. The resulting dryness, blotches and rosy patches require careful management. Look for products especially designed for sensitive skins – these will not contain perfume and irritants. Time and patience taken over the selection of skin-care and beauty products really does pay off. Specialized products cost no more but do contain active ingredients to keep sensitive skin comfortable and protected from harmful irritants and the elements. Do not use soap and water or facial washes on delicate skin, as they strip out moisture and oils, making the skin even more sensitive. Choose a light, unperfumed cleansing lotion, followed by a splash of warm water to remove any excess lotion. Avoid toners too, as they dry the skin, so causing further problems. Use a creamy moisturizer specially designed for dry, sensitive skin, and be sure to apply it both morning and night for the maximum benefit.

HOW DOES SKIN AGE?

Ten per cent of skin ageing is intrinsic, being dependent on your genes. Look at your parents: how has their skin fared as they've got older? They are a good indicator of how you might expect your skin to age. Eventually everyone looks older, but some age sooner than others.

Other factors – extrinsic, or lifestyle, factors – such as smoking, stress, bad diet and the weather can literally leave their mark in the form of lines, sags and wrinkles. The good news, though, is that you can take charge and choose which ones are going to affect your skin's ageing by being careful about exposing yourself to the sun, never smoking, sleeping well, eating healthily and avoiding toxins and pollutants.

Protect skin from the sun

Up to 80 per cent of premature ageing is caused by overexposure to the sun's harmful ultraviolet rays: a completely preventable source of ageing. Sun damage causes collagen and elastin to degenerate, as a result of which the skin sags and takes on a leathery appearance and texture, age spots develop and coarse wrinkles and broken blood vessels appear on the skin's surface. Sun damage over the years can develop into skin cancer, which may stay invisible for 20 years or more. For all these reasons it is vital that you protect your skin, especially the skin on your face, with a sunscreen containing a minimum sun protection factor of 15 (SPF15). (Note that, because of the way in which sunscreen works, it is never necessary to use a higher factor than SPF30, whatever the conditions.)

Stop smoking

As well as polluting your body with thousands of toxins, smoking takes its toll on the skin. As a result, smokers age badly. Smoking promotes the formation of free radicals in the body, which affect skin renewal at a cellular level, as well as restricting the circulation to many areas of the body, thereby starving the skin of the vital oxygen and nutrients it needs for a healthy complexion. Many smokers develop lines that run

from their mouth to their nose and have hollow cheeks from the inhaling motion. If that's not enough to put you off smoking, the fact that it also discolours the skin, hair and nails might be.

Steer clear of toxins

Toxins found in polluted air, drugs, pesticides, food and food additives, and chemicals are eliminated from the body by the liver, kidneys and lymph system. Good skin depends on healthy blood getting to the dermis and filtering the toxic waste away. An insufficient blood supply or blood high in toxins or

FREE RADICALS UNCOVERED

Free radicals are the destructive oxygen molecules that can accelerate the ageing process by breaking down the connective tissue, thinning skin and attacking muscle. Free radicals are very unstable and react quickly with other compounds; they tend to attack the nearest stable molecule to stabilize themselves, but in the process create another free radical. Once the process starts, it's a chain reaction ending with the disruption of a living cell.

Some free radicals arise normally during metabolism. Sometimes the body's immune system's cells create them to neutralize viruses and bacteria. The body can handle free radicals if it has a supply of antioxidants available. But if supplies run low or there is excessive free-radical production, then damage is the only outcome. Furthermore, free-radical damage accumulates with age. (See pages 20–21 for more information.)

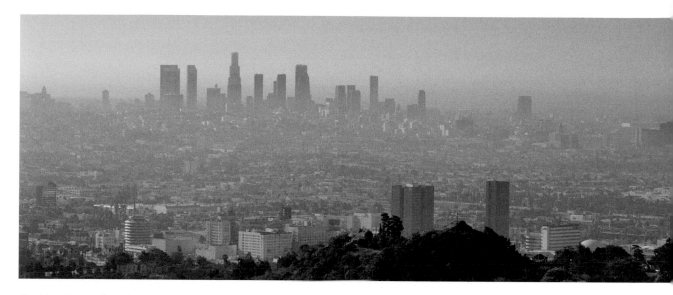

City life takes its toll on the skin, so if you are regularly exposed to polluted air, make efforts to detoxify your body.

accumulated waste undernourishes and overloads our systems. The skin then becomes a dumping ground for excess unfiltered toxins, which produce free radicals (see box). As a result of toxic overload, we often see deep furrows between the eyes and puffy under-eye bags. But the solution lies in your hands: steer clear of toxins in the first place, boost your circulation and detoxify your body.

Get a good night's sleep

We need beauty sleep so that our faces and bodies can relax and de-stress. Go to bed with a clean face for eight hours' sleep to give your skin cells the chance to regenerate. A lack of refreshing sleep or any kind of sleep deprivation shows itself as saggy eyelids, bags under the eyes and dark under-eye circles, along with a pallid complexion. Keep your bedroom well ventilated and not too dry, otherwise your skin's moisture will evaporate during the night, giving you dry skin.

Showing your age

In our thirties, damage from the sun, pollutants, bad diet and misuse of alcohol make skin changes more noticeable. The epidermis shows signs of wear and tear: you develop an uneven, dull complexion and fluid retention. The stratum corneum thickens as cell turnover begins to slow, and therefore the skin becomes less elastic and unable to bounce back. Facial expressions become etched into wrinkles, and this is when we start an interest in anti-ageing products.

As we progress through our forties, cell production takes longer and the basal layer (where new cells are made) and the epidermis become thinner. Cells begin to lose their ability to hold water, as a result of which the skin becomes more dry and sensitive. The stratum corneum thickens even more, sebum production declines and more dead cells accumulate on the surface, causing uneven pigmentation. It is at this time that thread veins appear on the scene.

Through our fifties, the menopause and the subsequent drop in oestrogen levels results in lower sebum production. With less oil available to protect the skin, more water evaporates from the surface, resulting in dry, flaky skin. The epidermis is now 20 per cent thinner than in the teenage years, and sun damage may appear as dark patches. Lower-level tissues have unevenly distributed cells, less collagen and elastin, allowing excess fat to form into deep furrows and droopy jowls.

Ageing, like everything in life, is subject to the forces of gravity, which means that everything eventually starts dropping. Throughout our sixties and seventies, we shrink as our bones naturally lose their bone mass. The skin around our bones sags and our muscles get thinner (increasingly so if they are not used regularly). Weight loss causes the face to look longer, particularly around the jowls, eyelids and the nose. Skin becomes increasingly dry, often paper thin, with age spots, blemishes and unevenly distributed pigmentation.

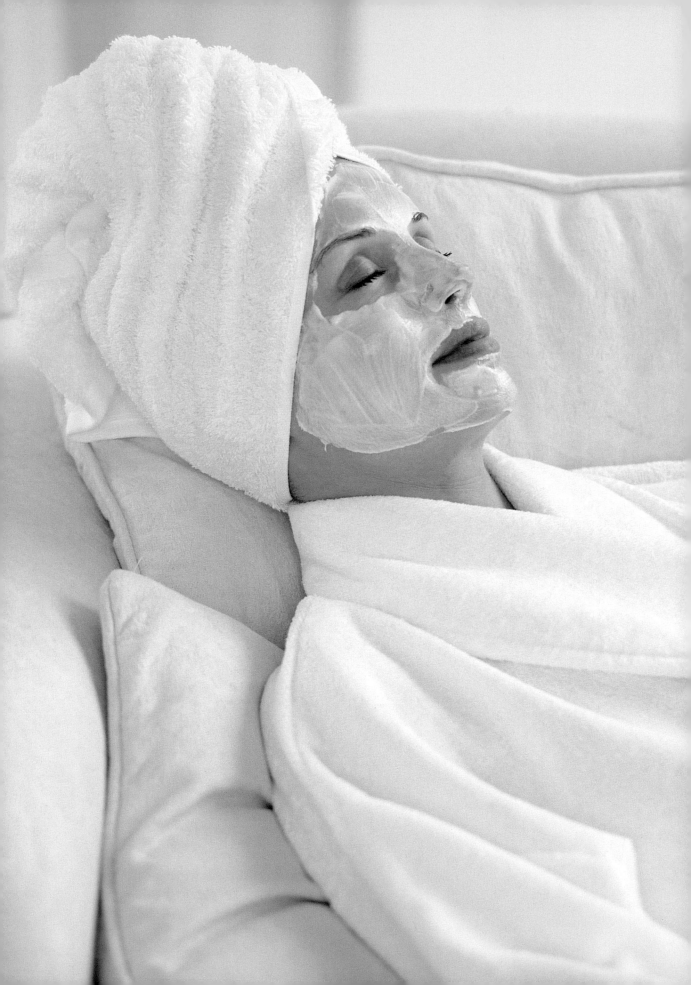

Instant beauty

Your skin is your body's largest organ, and what troubles it most are age and damage from the sun. New commercial skin-care and beauty products appear on the market daily, making fantastic promises to restore youthful skin. But can you revitalize and improve your skin? And are the products worth the money? Could home-made alternatives do the job at a fraction of the cost? Find out how simple tricks and techniques can enhance your natural beauty.

ESSENTIAL SKIN CARE

Maybe your skin is sensitive to the sun, your small blood capillaries are close to the surface or you have an oily skin? Whatever your assets or problems, try to nourish and maintain your skin for optimum beauty. Beauty is ageless: it just depends on knowing what your skin needs.

Cleansing

For skin to be healthy it needs to be clean, but too much washing is unnecessary and speeds up moisture loss from your skin. You could wash off the day's grime with water alone if you don't wear make-up; make-up wearers will need a cleanser to dissolve and remove not only the make-up but also the pollutants and bacteria that stick to it.

There are cleansers to suit all types of skin and pockets – including wash-off gels, foaming cleansers, wipe-away creams and milks, super-fatted soaps, soap-free beauty bars, dermatologic bars, antibacterial washes and instant cleansing wipes.

When choosing a cleanser, the general rule is to use a creamier cleanser on dry or more mature skin, a wipe-away lotion on normal skin and a wash-away cleanser on oilier skin. Of course, it is possible to find creamy washes and very drying lotion types, so experiment until you find one that suits your skin; ask for trial sizes at beauty counters. Also bear in mind that certain items of make-up, such as waterproof mascara, need special cleansers. And while wipes are convenient for travelling, late nights or emergencies, they shouldn't replace a good routine.

CLEANSING: APPLICATION

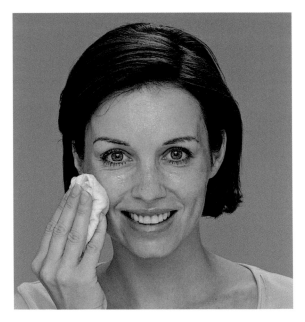

Apply wipe-away cleanser with fingers, leave for 30 seconds to dissolve make-up, then wipe gently away. Massage wash-away cleanser gently on skin, rinse thoroughly, finishing with several cold-water rinses.

GET INTO A ROUTINE

To maximize your skin's beauty potential, establish a good skin-care routine – morning and night.

Morning routine
- Cleanse to refresh your skin.
- Tone to remove any traces of creamy cleanser, unless you have oily skin.
- Moisturize to prevent further dryness and irritation, by locking in existing moisture and oils.

Night-time routine
- Cleanse thoroughly to remove all make-up and the grime from the day.
- Moisturize to feed your skin while you sleep.

Toning

You need to use a toner only after using a creamy cleanser, when you might need to remove excess oil and pore-clogging residue. Never use toner on an oily skin, as application only stimulates the skin more, making it oilier. Alcohol-based toners are too drying for most skins.

Make a simple rose-water toner for dry to normal skin by putting 100 ml (3½ fl oz) rose-water, 1 drop lavender oil and 1 drop frankincense in a small jar, shaking it well, then dabbing it on your face with a cotton wool pad. For normal to oily skin, use the same quantities of orange flower water, bergamot oil and cypress oil.

Moisturizing

Whichever formulation you choose, moisturizers help to prevent skin moisture loss. There is a fairly bewildering range on the market, but they split into three main categories:

- **Day creams** – these contain more water than oil and act to protect skin; they particularly suit oily skins.
- **Night creams** – these are richer and more oil-heavy, to feed sensitive and/or dry skin.
- **Lotions** – these tend to be oil-free and particularly suit combination skin types.

Your moisturizer must suit your lifestyle as well as your skin type, and may need to vary with the seasons. Unless you regularly exfoliate or polish your skin (see page 24), there is little point in using moisturizer, because a barrier of accumulated product and dead skin cells stops moisturizer getting through.

TIME OUT!

Give your skin an occasional break. Don't use any moisturizer or apply make-up and clean only with water plus a mild cleansing bar. Your natural skin will reveal itself after a week. Moisturizer may have caused clogged pores, foundation may have resulted in some irritation and the wrong toner may have dried out your skin.

TONING: APPLICATION

MOISTURIZING: APPLICATION

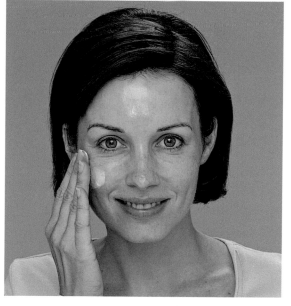

After cleansing, rinse your face with warm water, or a pad soaked with toner, then gently pat or stroke your skin clean, avoiding sensitive eye areas.

Finally, apply moisturizer, particularly around the eyes, where there are fewer sebaceous glands. Rub it in lightly, using a circular motion. Always allow moisturizer to soak in before applying make-up.

MIRACLE INGREDIENTS

Years of cosmetic research and development are paying off with the arrival of new and innovative skin-care products. Experiment with the latest proven anti-ageing ingredients (the cheaper products as well as the expensive, highly packaged ones) to find out if they work for you.

Alpha-hydroxy acids

These acidic substances claim to have an abrasive, exfoliating effect that sloughs off dead surface skin cells and encourages the cellular cycle. They are water soluble, boost water retention and plump up skin, thereby giving it a more youthful appearance. Alpha-hydroxy acids (known as AHAs) are found naturally in unripened fruit, milk and sugar cane. They include lactic acid (milk), glycolic acid (sugar cane), citric acid (citrus and molasses), malic acid (apples) and tartaric acid (grapes). Other acids are manufactured synthetically to mimic these naturally occurring ones. Many people are allergic to AHAs, and others experience skin photosensitivity when wearing them, making it essential to wear sunscreen protection too. Some moisturizers contain AHAs and SPF.

Beta-hydroxy acids

Beta-hydroxy acids (BHAs) are exfoliants and claim to be potent anti-agers, reducing the appearance of wrinkles and uneven, patchy skin pigmentation. They are less abrasive than AHAs and slightly lighter, which makes them more suitable for sensitive skins; they are also effective on oily skin for blackheads and whiteheads. The BHA used in cosmetic products, which is derived from willow bark (salicylic acid), was originally used as a peeling agent to treat acne. These acids can also cause skin photosensitivity, so if your products contain them, be sure to wear some sunscreen during the day.

Retinoids

These anti-ageing ingredients are derived from vitamin A; examples include retinol, retinyl palmatate and tretinoin. Originally used as an acne treatment, they work by unplugging pores, so enabling the skin's natural oil, sebum, to surface more quickly. Under the surface, retinoids help to rejuvenate the skin by encouraging the formation of collagen and elastin, both of which deplete as we grow older, leading to less elastic skin. Users of these products report less-obvious lines and wrinkles. Retinoids can cause stinging, redness and light sensitivity, so use sunscreen with any products that contain them.

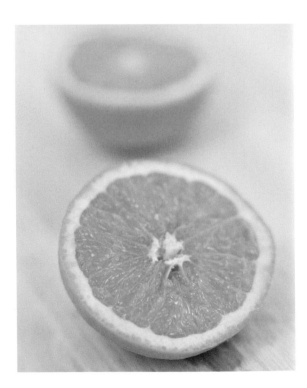

Citric acid, which is extracted from oranges and other citrus fruits or made by fermenting molasses, is one of the alpha-hydroxy acids found in many skin-care products.

ANTIOXIDANT PROTECTION

As we age, the body begins to form highly reactive chemicals called free radicals, which attack cells and oxidize flesh, scrambling the molecular make-up of skin and other tissues and starving the cells of vital oxygen. The main victim, as far as your face is concerned, is collagen: the results of the free-radical damage are a tough, leathery skin. By the age of 50, it is estimated that 30 per cent of the body's cellular protein has been damaged by free-radical activity. The results are wrinkles, under-eye bags and creases.

Fortunately the best weapon against free radicals is a certain type of nutrient that occurs naturally in many foods – antioxidants. These nutrients can slow down the oxidizing process and keep your skin looking younger for longer.

More than 100 antioxidants have been identified, but the main ones are betacarotene; vitamins A, C and E; selenium and zinc. Vitamins C and E and betacarotene are most effective if taken together, as they work in synergy. Other antioxidants include bioflavonoids, proanthocyanidins and anthocyanidins. Copper and magnesium may be taken as supplements.

Betacarotene is the plant form of vitamin A, which the body converts into vitamin A. It protects against the effects of ultraviolet light, boosts the body's natural immunity and can protect the skin from bacterial infection. Betacarotene is a carotenoid; others include lutein, zeaxanthine and lycopene.

Vitamin A improves skin texture.

Vitamin C has a reputation for being the most potent antioxidant. It is also essential for the production of collagen, the elastic tissue in skin that declines with age. Boosting your vitamin C intake may slow down loss of collagen.

Vitamin E is probably the best-known skin nutrient. As an antioxidant, it works in tandem with selenium and has the most powerful action against free-radical damage caused by the sun. It also helps the skin to retain moisture, to maximize its use of oxygen and to produce new cells where the skin has been damaged.

Selenium protects cells from free radicals and helps to counter dry skin. Along with vitamin E, it supports the immune system so it can help to fight infection.

Zinc, like vitamin C, is vital to the manufacture of collagen. It speeds up the healing process where skin has been damaged, and evens out pigmentation. It is vital to the immune system, and so helps to destroy infection. A lack of zinc slows down skin healing and can lead to stretch marks and stubborn blemishes.

Bioflavonoids are a group of 500 compounds or more, some of which are potent antioxidants. They work with vitamin C to protect and condition connective tissue and capillaries.

Proanthocyanidins and anthocyanidins are less well-known members of the antioxidant club, but they can still claim elite status. In addition to their own antioxidant activities, they enhance the antioxidant powers of vitamins A, C and E. They are also believed to inhibit the enzymes responsible for the breakdown of elastin and collagen in the connective tissue. Some particularly potent forms, known as oligomeric proanthocyanidins, are gradually being incorporated into skin creams, but they can also be consumed in green tea, turmeric and grape seeds.

Coenzyme Q10 helps skin repair itself and is an effective free-radical fighter.

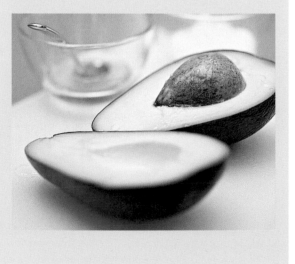

A WEEKLY FACIAL

Some skin-care routines are best done just once, or maybe twice, a week. Once you have exfoliated your skin using one of the scrub recipes shown here, you need to rehydrate it afterwards. For some self-indulgent skin care, try a facial mask, tonic or feed.

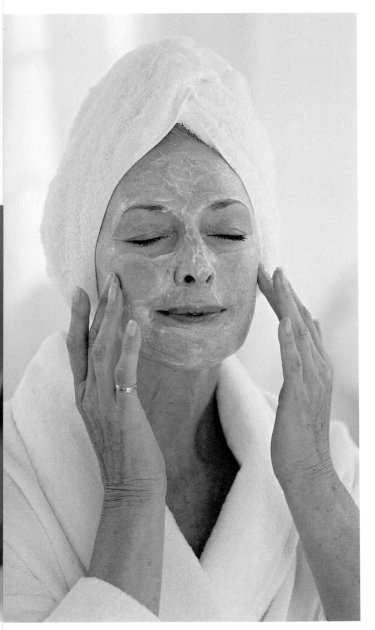

Exfoliating

Dead skin cells and surplus grime make your skin look dull and prevent helpful products from penetrating the skin. So, once a week after routine cleansing, exfoliate (or 'polish') your skin to get it thoroughly clean. Exfoliating creams contain tiny scrubbing grains to slough off dead surface cells and stimulate the skin's natural renewal process. Simply dampen your skin with water, and then apply the cream, using your fingertips to make very light, small, circular movements. Massage both the skin and the underlying muscles in an upward direction to improve blood circulation and encourage lymphatic drainage. Avoid the delicate eye area, where the skin is too fine for this exfoliating treatment, but don't neglect your neck (unless your skin is particularly sensitive there). Massage for 1–2 minutes, and then rinse off the cream with tepid water.

Many exfoliating creams contain natural ground ingredients including apricot kernels, which are too harsh for sensitive skins. Others contain synthetic, round, evenly shaped scrubbing grains, which are kinder to delicate skin. For the homespun approach, you could exfoliate your entire body with used coffee grounds in the shower or with fine sand by the sea. Alternatively, you could try making your own scrub recipes at home (see opposite page).

Rehydrating

Once you have exfoliated your skin, you should moisturize it immediately while it is still damp so

Once a week, give you skin a thorough polish, with a gentle, exfoliating massage. Choose from a selection of commercial creams or make your own.

HOME-MADE FACIAL SCRUBS

Scrubs are used to exfoliate, or polish, your skin, and these home-produced ones are cheap to make.

Oat nut scrub

2 tsp fine oatmeal
2 tsp ground almonds
orange flower water (for oily skin) or cream
    (for dry skin) to blend

Sugar corn scrub

2 tsp cornflower
2 tsp raw brown sugar
1 tsp almond oil
apple juice (for normal skin) or lemon juice
    (for oily skin) to blend

Sticky grape scrub

2 tsp salt
1 dsp grape juice
Greek yogurt to blend

Whichever scrub you want to make, mix the ingredients into a smooth paste then leave for 5 minutes to bind. Gently massage into the face, avoiding the delicate skin under the eyes. Wipe off with a damp muslin cloth (more gentle than a face cloth), rinse your face in warm water then gently pat dry with a towel.

that you lock in the water remaining on your skin. Skin dehydration is exacerbated by central heating, air conditioning, wind and the sun. To counter the drying effect of central heating, place a humidifier in your bedroom or a pan of water on a radiator, and take short baths in warm water, adding oils to prevent dry, cracking skin. Skin needs water to be healthy, and hydrating face masks, such as the avocado and honey recipe provided here, can help enormously. To attain maximum hydration, drink less coffee, tea and alcohol (all of which have a dehydrating effect), or at least change to decaff versions, and drink more plain water. Aim for a daily quota of six to eight glasses of water – freshly squeezed fruit juices and herbal infusions count too.

HOME-MADE FACIAL NUTRITION

A mask, a tonic and a nutritious feed will all do wonders for your skin.

Avocado and honey nourishing mask

The rich oils in avocado, the humectant quality of honey and the stimulating effects of these essential oils make this a good feed for dry, ageing skin.

quarter of a ripe avocado
1 tsp runny honey
2 tsp live Greek yogurt
2 drops jasmine or rose otto

Mash the avocado very thoroughly with a fork, then stir in the remaining ingredients. Apply quite thickly to the face and leave on for at least 10 minutes. Wipe off with a dry muslin cloth, then rinse the cloth in warm water and use it to remove the rest of the mask. After such a rich mask, it is a good idea to perk up your skin with a refreshing toner, such as the rose-water recipe on page 19.

Cucumber and clay tonic

The astringent properties of cucumber and clay make this a good tonic for normal to oily skin.

5 cm (2 inch) piece of cucumber
4 tsp green clay
2 tsp brewer's yeast

Put all the ingredients in a blender and mix until smooth. If the mixture is a little watery, add another teaspoon or two of clay.

Turmeric and egg feed

The essential fats in the egg yolk and the softening properties of turmeric make this a luxurious facial feed for tired and dry to normal skin.

1 egg, separated   2 tsp turmeric
2 tsp brewer's yeast   2 tsp pollen grains
2 dsp jojoba oil   rose-water to blend

Whisk the egg yolk and then add the remaining ingredients. This feed is easy to apply but rather sticky, so sponge it off carefully. It will leave your skin feeling beautifully smooth.

LYMPHATIC DRAINAGE

The lymphatic drainage system eliminates waste and toxins, and this lymphatic massage will help to kickstart sluggish systems, which cause grey pallor, tired eyes and puffy skin.

Promoting drainage

Massaging the soft tissue and muscle greatly speeds up the lymphatic elimination process. A short weekly session will rid the body of any unwanted waste products that have escaped routine elimination by the body's detoxification systems. The aim of a lymphatic drainage massage is to direct toxins to the nearest lymph node for dispersal. You can work on the lymph areas around your shoulders and head, to eliminate any puffiness around your face and under-eye bags and to improve your complexion.

Sadly, much of the toxic accumulation could be caused by your lifestyle: if you are lazy or simply have a very sedentary job, your lymph will not be pumped around your system, and so will not do the eliminating job it was designed for.

LYMPHATIC DRAINAGE MASSAGE

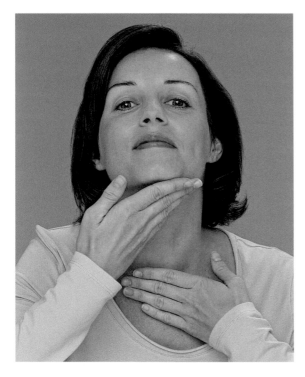

1 Rub 1 tsp oil on to your hands. With sweeping movements, slide your hands from your chest to your chin upwards from the left side of your neck, lightly over your windpipe and then to the right.

2 Place your first fingers horizontally above your lips, with your middle fingers below. Apply a slight pressure and then slide your fingers backwards to your ears.

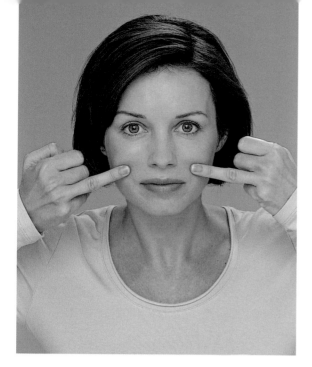

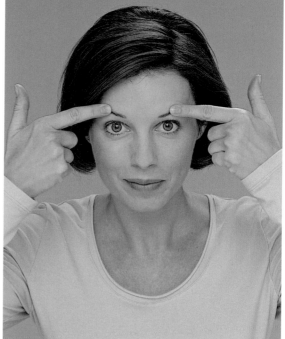

3 Place your ring fingers by the side of each nostril and apply pressure. Release the pressure as you sweep your fingers across your cheeks to your ears, then reapply the pressure.

4 Place your first fingers in the centre of your forehead. Pressing firmly, slide your fingers as you trace along your eyebrows and out to your ears.

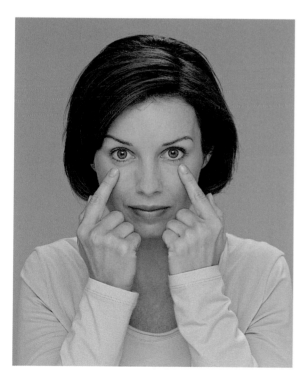

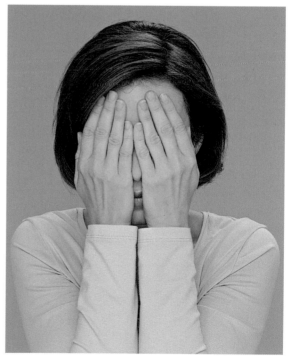

5 Now, from your ears, continue sliding your fingertips lightly, tracing inwards under the eyes to your nose.

6 Close your eyes and cover your entire face, from chin to forehead (leave your nose protruding) with your open hands. Press your whole face firmly, hold for 5 seconds and then release.

EMERGENCY QUICK-FIXES

Whether your skin needs a moisture boost or a deep cleanse, whether your eyes are puffy or red, or whether you just can't seem to get rid of dry lips, many of these emergency remedies can be made in your own home for instant quick-fixing.

Use face masks for instant results

For a simple 'pick-me-up' apply any of the following face masks, to suit your skin type, after exfoliating. Using a face mask as a weekly treat for your skin will certainly show results.

- To rescue sensitive skin, use this moist cucumber mask, which won't harden and is easily removed. Simply mash half a cucumber and apply to your skin. Leave for 15 minutes, then wash off with cool water.

  Another treatment suitable for sensitive skin is chamomile, which is anti-inflammatory. Use over-the-counter chamomile lotion to calm and de-stress delicate skin that has been reddened by exfoliating.

- To feed dry skin, treat it to a weekly gelatine mask. To 125 ml (4 fl oz) of apple juice, add a packet of unflavoured gelatine. Heat and mix (microwave for 30 seconds), leave it to cool, then put it in the fridge to set. When it is cold, spread it over your face, leave for 15 minutes, then rinse off with cool water.

- To pep-up normal skin, apply an invigorating grape mask once or twice a week. Simply mash six grapes and mix with a teaspoon of cornflour. Pat on to your face, and leave to dry for 15 minutes. Use warm water to remove it, followed by some cold water.

- To tone normal and combination skins, use a yogurt mask, which tones and tightens the skin while drawing out bacteria and oil. Mix 2 teaspoonfuls of brewer's yeast with 60 ml (2 fl oz) of plain yogurt, and add a teaspoon of wine vinegar. Apply the mask to your face, and leave for 15 minutes. Wash off with tepid water.

- To detox oily skin, use a clay or mud mask to absorb oils and draw out impurities. Apply, leave to harden for 15 minutes, then remove with tepid water. Masks containing wheat, corn or charcoal will all efficiently dry up oils.

Calm puffy eyes

Puffy eyes can mean that you've used too much eye cream. During sleep, body heat melts any cream on the face and it can slide into the eye itself. To avoid getting eye cream in your eye, simply apply a small

TOP TIPS FOR GREAT-LOOKING SKIN

- Wake up tired-looking skin by massaging it with moisturizer (morning or night) for 5 minutes.
- Give tired-looking skin an instant bloom by using moisturizers, foundations and balms that contain light-diffusing properties.
- For special occasions, paint egg white over lined areas on droopy faces. It temporarily tightens and lifts the face. Allow it to dry completely before applying any make-up.
- Lighten age spots on hands and face with lemon juice, though note that this treatment is not suitable for sensitive skin.

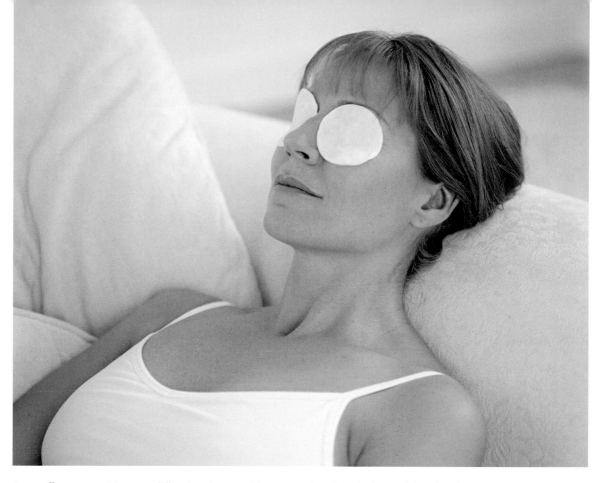

Treat puffy eyes to a 10-minute chill-out by placing cold cotton wool pads soaked in witch hazel on them.

amount and lightly tap it along your eye socket bone (2.5 cm/1 inch below your eye) with your fingertips. During the night, the cream will travel in fine lines to all the eye areas.

Puffy eyes are also a sign of poor blood and lymph circulation and can indicate lack of sleep, tiredness, excess consumption of alcohol or stress. To counter these puffy eyes, place used, cold tea bags, cucumber slices, cotton wool pads soaked in witch hazel or two metal teaspoons (all kept in the fridge) on to closed eyes. Relax for 10 minutes.

Soothe red eyes

Spending time in smoky environments can make your eyes red, itchy and uncomfortable. Calm them with cotton wool pads soaked in cold milk, then placed on closed eyes for 10 minutes. Milk has an anti-inflammatory effect and soothes the redness.

You can use eye drops to brighten red eyes and temporarily shrink the blood vessels, but these are quick-fix solutions only and should not be relied on for daily treatment. If you are concerned about your eyes, make an appointment for an eye examination.

Banish dark circles

Whether they are due to poor circulation of blood or an accumulation of toxins under the thin surface skin (possibly from excess alcohol, cigarettes or coffee), you can remedy dark circles in two ways. Place two thin slices of raw potato on top of closed eyes for 10 minutes and relax. Alternatively, become more active – take a brisk walk, do facial exercises and get your lymphatic drainage system moving (see pages 26–27).

Get rid of under-eye bags

Although these are often hereditary, you can boost the lymphatic and blood circulations to counter these bags. If they persist, use a darker shade of matt concealer to help disguise them. To kickstart the circulation, simply tap your fingertips along your lower eye socket, from the inside corner to the outer eye.

Reverse lip dryness

If your lips are dry, stop licking them. As the saliva evaporates, it destroys the lips' natural protection and makes them drier. Fragile lip skin doesn't contain oil glands, so use lip balm under lipstick to moisturize it.

TRICKS OF THE TRADE

You can instantly help yourself to a younger look and brighter complexion simply by updating the way you apply your make-up. Make-up artists are skilled in the knowledge of how to make the most of people's faces, and now you can benefit from their experience.

As we get older, we all suffer the same fate: blemishes appear, the fine lines become wrinkles, and the skin loses its bloom. But help is at hand in the form of the 'tricks of the trade' of make-up artists, who use colour to enhance assets and disguise faults.

Take a long, good look
What are your good and bad points? Remove your make-up (if you wear it), scrape your hair back and,

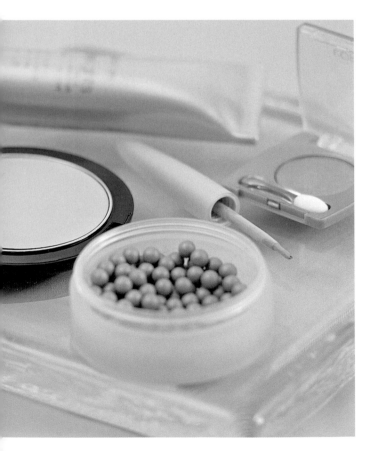

in a good light, take a long, hard look at yourself. Be honest, and don't focus just on things you don't like about yourself, or you won't see a thing! Scrutinize your face, giving yourself credit for your good points that you really can see in the mirror today (not to be confused with what you used to see some years ago). Be positive in your approach – only then can you learn to emphasize your good points, rather than just hiding your bad ones.

Changing times
Remember how, when you were young, you wanted to wear make-up to appear grown up? Today, many mature women still apply the same colours and techniques they experimented with 20 or 30 years ago, and still manage to make themselves appear older. Make-up artists and beauty consultants can judge a woman's age from the way she wears her make-up. Some mature women can easily rely on old favourites and may not change their products, colours or application since first trying things out as a teenager. When correctly applied, make-up can take five or 10 years off your face, but how? The idea to remember is that good make-up is one that looks good for you, regardless of fashion, brand or price.

Make-up is a godsend when it comes to hiding signs of fatigue. Over recent years, beauty scientists have designed cosmetics specifically for weary skin. Now, light-reflecting pigments are included in foundations, blushers and eye shadows to brighten the face and put lines and blemishes into soft focus: a boon for mature skin.

Try some of the new products available today to see if you could update your make-up bag and improve your look.

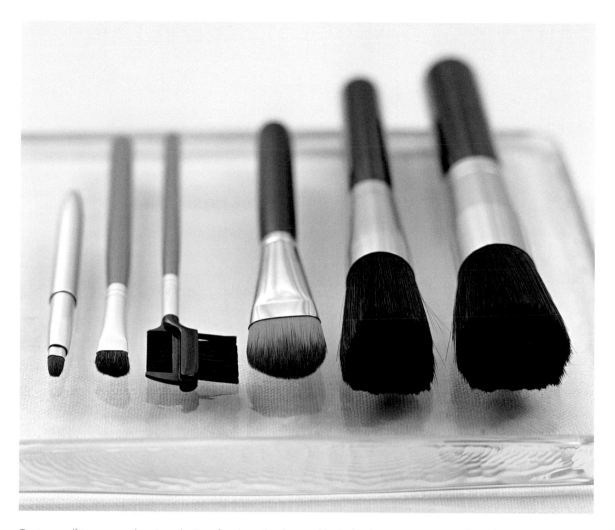

Treat yourself to a comprehensive selection of make-up brushes, and look after them to ensure years of good use.

The right tools for the job

The saying 'A bad workman always blames his tools' is just as applicable to make-up as it is to carpentry. If you use poor-quality brushes or applicators (the type that come with eye shadows or blushers, which can be scratchy and hard to control), you will almost certainly produce bad results. So treat yourself to some new brushes – the best quality you can afford – and, if you look after them, they will last for years.

Small, good-quality, sable artist's brushes are excellent for applying eye shadow, eyeliner and lipsticks, while a large round brush of good quality, the fattest possible, is ideal for blusher. A combined eyelash brush and eyebrow comb brushes out excess mascara, separates your eyelashes and gives the finishing touch to well-shaped eyebrows. To keep brushes in tip-top shape, wash them weekly with mild shampoo, swish in clear water, blot, shape and then stand upright overnight in a mug to dry.

Brushes stay in condition if you keep them upright, clean and in shape. When travelling, use the inside of a toilet roll to protect big blusher brushes and a straw for smaller brushes.

THE GOLDEN RULE FOR SKIN

Whether you wear lots, little or no make-up at all, remember one golden rule: protect your skin from pollution, the elements and particularly the sun. Choose those skin-care creams and gels that contain a minimum of SPF15.

WHAT'S YOUR FACE SHAPE?

Now's the time to use the 'tricks of the trade' to Define, Enhance, Conceal, Improve, Detract and Experiment on your looks. DECIDE how to make the most of your face, and enjoy the results.

All of us look quite different from one another, and, unless we have cosmetic surgery, our basic features are likely to remain pretty much the same throughout our lives. We spend time and money on products to improve the quality of our skin, but so often ruin our good work by applying our make-up badly.

Work with your face shape

First, get to know your face a bit better, and take a careful look at – and also feel – your facial features.

- Sit in front of a mirror in a good light. Remove all your make-up (if you wear it), tie or clip back your hair and close your eyes.
- Now open your eyes wide and look quickly at your face (as though you were a stranger); objectively analyse what you see.
- Feel your cheekbones with your fingertips, and lightly walk them along your cheekbones to your ears. Now smile, determine and feel the 'apple' – that fleshy mound of flesh in the middle of your cheeks.
- Lightly trace around the edge of your lips with your fingertips, becoming aware of their border; this is where you will draw your lip line.
- Close your eyes and put your forefingers on your eyelids, next to your lashes; this is where you will put on eyeliner.
- Gently feel the curve of your eyeballs through your eyelids; use a neutral or basic colour eye shadow here.
- Moving your forefingers up, place them under your eyebrows on the eye socket bone and open your eyes wide. Here, and in the centre top of your eyebrow, is where you will put highlighter.
- If you feel straggly eyebrows above, maybe they need tidying up a little.

Once you have established your bone structure and know your face, applying make-up is that bit easier. The choice is yours, DECIDE and have fun.

The five basic face shapes

Despite skin colour and age, most faces fall into five basic shapes. Within these basic shapes are the individual features that give each of us our unique looks.

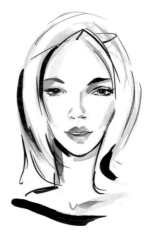

1 Oval-shaped face

This face shape is often seen as classic beauty, with balanced, evenly spaced features.

- Apply blusher to the apple of the cheek for a healthy, younger look.
- Define the lips or eyes and emphasize the best features.
- Pair strong eyes with strong lips.
- Match bare, pale eyes with muted lips.

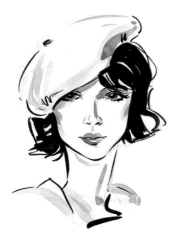

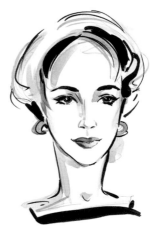

2 Heart-shaped face

With a wider forehead curving down to a point, a heart-shaped face has dainty features.

- Add blusher to the hollows just under the cheekbones.
- Highlight the chin tip with pale/ivory-coloured powder (or eye shadow).
- Add definition to the lips and eyes.

3 Long face

Often this face shape is narrow, with a deep forehead, high cheekbones and strong jaw.

- Start the blusher on the apple and brush it out to the sides: your face will appear wider and fresher.
- Don't emphasize the eyebrow arch but create a straighter line and taper it towards the ear tip.
- Keep the focus on lips and eyes; highlight the centre of the face by dusting the tip of the nose.

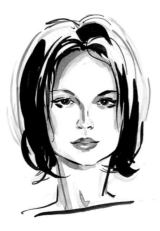

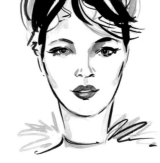

4 Square face

This face shape is a square with a soft appearance.

- Just brush a light colour on the apple; with your defined face shape you don't need much shaping.
- Softly highlight the centre strip (forehead, nose and chin tip) by dusting with ivory-coloured powder (or eye shadow).
- Slightly darken the face outline and jaw line using powder a shade darker than your normal.
- Focus on the lips and eyes.

5 Round face

This face shape is wide and short, with a smaller nose, round chin and full cheeks.

- Start the blusher midway from the apple, brushing upwards to the cheekbone to add definition.
- Softly highlight the chin.
- Create full cheeks, as they look youthful.
- Avoid overemphasizing the eyes with a heavy eyeliner.
- Use eye colour to elongate the eyes and so balance your face.

USING FOUNDATION

As we grow older, our skin, like our hair, becomes uneven and loses some of its colour, so it's important to keep changing the shade of your foundation with the years.

Foundation is designed to even out skin tones and hide slight blemishes. The trick is to use just the minimum amount, while still using enough to present a flawless, natural-looking complexion.

Applying foundation

For the best results, apply your foundation using a small, slightly damp cosmetic sponge with light feathery movements. Or, if you prefer, use your fingertips – the heat from your fingers helps with the blending. Sponges can absorb 60 per cent of foundation, so professional make-up artists often use a large brush instead.

Do not pile on the foundation. Rather than disguising the flaws, too much make-up accentuates them, because it collects into the lines on the face, adding years to your age. Also, avoid using foundation on very dry patches of skin: it will stick to them and make your skin look blemished and older. Finally, be careful not to add much foundation close to the eyes or lips if you have any lines. The powder will collect in the lines, widening and exaggerating them.

CHOOSING YOUR FOUNDATION

Look for a foundation that exactly matches your skin tone. Test the colour by running a small amount along the jaw line – it should virtually disappear. You can always mix two colours to achieve just the right blend or to make your base a little lighter or darker, according to the season.

Older skins respond well to lightweight, sheer foundations, which add luminosity. If your foundation seems a little heavy, try diluting it with moisturizer or adding some sunscreen for extra protection.

Problem areas

Flushed cheeks, veins, spots, under-eye bags and puffiness need a little extra cover. Use a matching concealer, or a layer of dried-out foundation from around the tube top, applied with a small, clean lip brush or tiny sponge. Tap your fingers lightly around the edges to blend in, but don't use your fingers to cover spots because you risk spreading bacteria.

APPLYING FOUNDATION

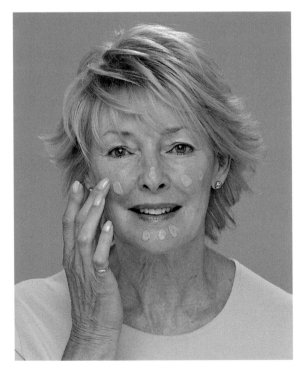

1 Cleanse and moisturize your face and neck before applying foundation. Then dab small amounts of the foundation that best matches your skin colour on to your cheeks, nose, chin and forehead.

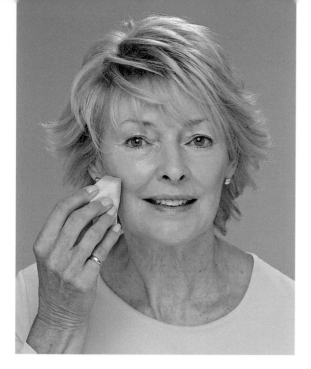

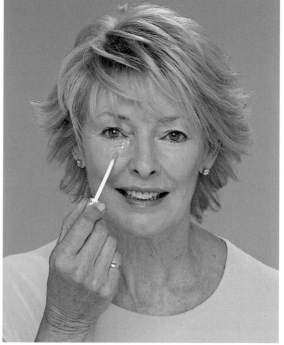

2 Blend the foundation outwards from the T-zone of the nose and eyes, using light, feathery movements. Blend down to just under your jaw line and out to your hairline.

3 Add brightness to tired under-eye areas with a 'magic wand' concealer, which contains light-reflecting pigments. Stroke the wand down from your inner eyes to the top of your cheek.

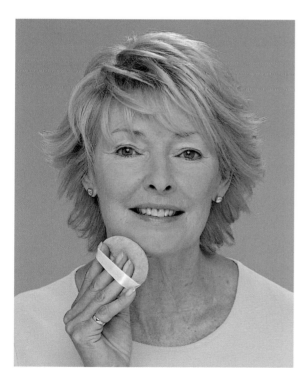

4 Dust your face all over with a little translucent face powder to achieve that all-important matt finish to your make-up. (If your face becomes shiny during the day, retouch with some more powder.)

5 Finally, press a dampened sponge all over your face. This creates a natural look by settling the powder, which then stays in place and, more importantly, looks good all day.

ADDING COLOUR

We all have days when our tired and washed-out faces could do with a pick-me-up, colour-wise. But you can also use blusher to do more than just give your cheeks a rosy glow.

Blusher adds a warm glow and helps define your face, but if your cheeks are naturally rosy, you could skip blusher altogether. Too much blusher can age your face: it settles in wrinkles, drawing attention to them. If you apply blusher before doing your eyes, you'll use less eye make-up and the effect will be more natural.

Powder blusher

The powdered form of blusher is the most popular and works well on all skin types, including oily skin. Apply before powdering, but remember that too matt a surface can emphasize wrinkles. Tap the brush on your hand before applying to avoid too much colour.

Cream blusher

This blusher formulation works well on normal and dry skin, but is not good for oily skins. Cream blushers are excellent for mature skins because there is less emphasis on lines, since there is no powder element to settle into them. If you don't like a powdered look, use cream blusher after applying foundation or mix with some tinted moisturizer for a fresh, dewy look. Apply by dotting the blusher along your cheekbones, then blend with your fingertips for a no-make-up, younger look. You don't have to stop at just your cheeks – apply cream blusher to your eyes and lips as well. Quick and easy for those on the go!

APPLYING POWDER BLUSHER

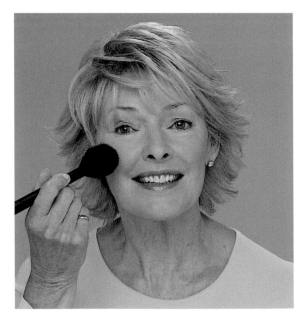

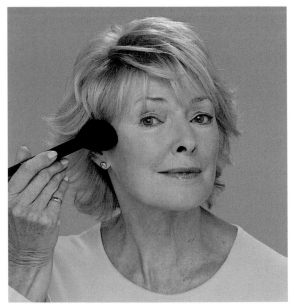

1 Stroke the blusher high on the apples of your cheeks; natural coral pink gives a young glow.

2 Continue the line of blusher out to the top of your cheekbone, where your ear meets your face.

Gel blusher

If you have oily skin, this light, sheer and transparent blusher is ideal for you. Usually waterproof, it's great for sports and a bare, natural look. It can be difficult to blend, especially on dry skin, so moisturize your face well before dotting this along your cheekbones.

Stick blusher

Somewhere in between a cream and a powder, stick blusher can be used on cheeks, lips and even as eye shadow. Although it is creamy to apply, once on your face it takes on a soft powdery look.

Bronzing blusher

If your skin is in good condition, or you have a light tan, use bronzing powder instead of blusher to extend your tan. For fair skins with a light tan, use soft, pinky bronze; darker skins can take deeper shimmering tones.

The perfect combination

For a long-lasting effect, apply cream blusher, tapping it along your cheekbones and smoothing it in. Set this with a little translucent powder, then go over your cheeks with powder blusher in a similar shade.

WHERE TO BLUSH?

The simplest way to find out where to place blusher is to smile at your reflection in the mirror. Apply blusher where your cheeks are plumpest (the apple) and blend towards your hairline (see also pages 32–33). For a young, natural look, the colour to choose is the colour that your cheeks go naturally when flushed. However, if your face is round, or you want to make your cheekbones more prominent, imagine a line from the top point of your cheekbone (where your ear meets your face) to the outer corner of your mouth, and run blusher along this line to halfway down your cheek. You could try placing a pencil along this line to act as a guide; you will find it sits under your cheekbone. Also use blusher to contour and sharpen your jaw line. Don't confine blusher to cheeks: use it to brush lightly around your hairline, or, for a quick eye lift, flick it lightly right across your eyelids. During summer months, try swapping your blusher for bronzing powder to give you a healthy look without having to expose yourself to the sun.

APPLYING CREAM BLUSHER

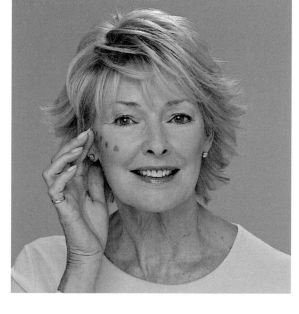

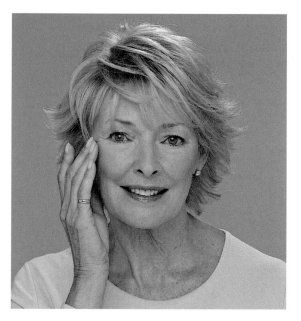

1 Dot the blusher along your cheekbone, following its contour as it curves upwards.

2 Gently blend the blusher with your foundation, so that just a subtle hint of colour is left.

YOUNGER EYES

The days of neutral and brown are over: make-up counters are now full of exciting rainbow colours. Select your colours confidently, but avoid using too much colour – it just isn't flattering. The subtle use of colours should attract attention to your eyes, but not overpower them.

To find which eye shadow, eyeliner and mascara colours suit you best, look closely at the iris of your eye. The iris has myriad coloured flecks, all individually suited to you. Which colour you choose is down to personal choice, though it is worth noting that a large splash of any colour across the lids is not flattering. Try experimenting with colours you do not normally use: you might just find the perfect one.

The colour for you

Applying the right colour can work wonders for a tired-looking face and make a dramatic difference to your looks. For example, silvery-grey, stone and pale pink eye shadows work well on mature eyelids, giving the face that required lift. Delicate skin around the eyes naturally loses elasticity with age; the resulting crepey skin needs to be treated carefully. Avoid drawing attention to it; concentrate your eye shadow on the lid, near to the lash line. Mature women should avoid eye shadows containing sparkle, as it draws attention to lines and can also irritate sensitive skin and eyes.

Line your eyes

Whether to outline your eyes for dramatic effect depends on your individuality, age or the occasion. But it's wise to avoid dramatic liquid eyeliner completely – unless you are 18. Instead, opt for a brown, grey or navy eyeliner or kohl; these colours are more flattering for a mature face than black.

Emphasize those lashes

Be selective when buying your mascara – it's best to leave the dramatic, fibre-enriched version for special occasions. If you use waterproof mascara, you will need a special eye make-up remover.

TOP TIPS FOR YOUR EYE SHAPE

- **Large, round** – *Eyelid*: medium or dark shadow from outer corner up, blended and continued over three-quarters of eyelid; lighter shade at inner corner. *Upper lash line*: complete line; *lower lash line*: from outside corner, one-third of the way only.
- **Small** – *Eyelid*: medium tone on outer corner of eyes, angled up, continued over entire eyelid up to crease, with darker colour from crease to outer corner. *Upper lash line*: complete line; *lower lash line*: from outer corner, one-third of the way only.
- **Close-set** – *Eyelid*: lighter shadow from inside corner, darker shadow on outside corner, extended up and out. Highlight under brow and outer eye corner. *Upper/lower lash lines*: from centre to outside corner.
- **Wide-set** – *Eyelid*: medium shadow from outside corner up over entire lid to crease; darker colour to emphasize inner corner and blend up to brow; lighter shade on centre of brow only. *Upper/lower lash lines*: complete lines.
- **Hooded** – *Eyelid*: medium shadow at outer corners, working up; dark shade over hooded area blended to brow; medium tone on lid, blended to brow; light shade to inside corner and high up under eyebrows. *Upper lash line*: complete line; *lower lash line*: from outside corner, one-third only.
- **Droopy** – *Eyelid*: medium shadow on outer corner, blended up; lighter shadow from inner corner, blended up; dark shadow at outside corner of crease and on centre lid. *Upper lash line*: stopping short of outer corner; *lower lash line*: from outside corner to three-quarters of the way only.

APPLYING EYELINER

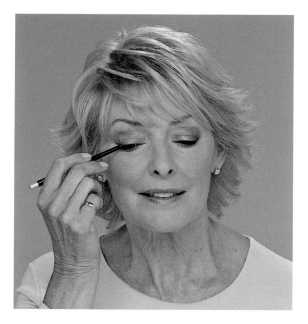

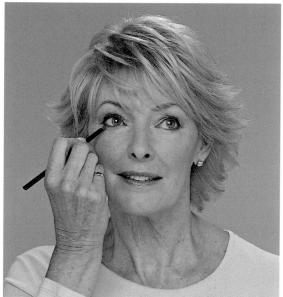

1 Using an eyeliner pencil or kohl, trace a line along the upper lash line, working from the inside corner outwards.

2 When working on the lower lash line, start from the outside corner, but end midway along to create a flattering, more open-eyed look.

APPLYING MASCARA

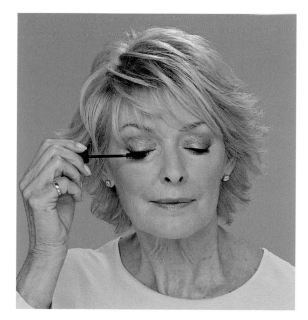

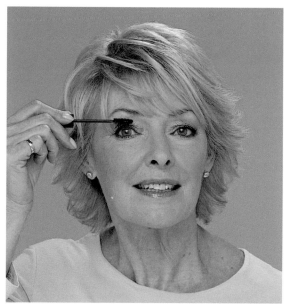

1 Start by brushing down over the top of your upper eyelashes, ideally using a grey mascara, which is more flattering than black for mature women.

2 Now brush the lashes up from underneath, looking straight at the mirror. Finally, add mascara sparingly to the lower lashes.

CHOOSING EYE COLOUR

Finding the right colour eye shadow is a case of trial and error, but it pays to keep experimenting until you do. Avoid the common mistake of matching a shadow to your eye colour or the colour of your outfit: instead go for something more colourful and eye-catching.

When choosing colours, it pays to look closely at the colours in your iris. Blue eyes aren't only blue: they are often flecked with grey, amber and green, so choose a shadow to match one of these colours. Note, though, that if the colour is too harsh it will dominate, making your natural eye colour dull by comparison. The paler your skin, the softer your colour needs to be, as intense colours will leave your eyes looking washed out. While brown eye shadow is safe and flatters all eye colours, try other colours for special occasions, but avoid any harsh lines. As with all make-up, the secret for a more youthful look is to blend well.

Colour choices for hazel and violet eyes

If your eyes are hazel, try eye shadow colours of grey, heather, olive, cocoa, apricot or peach.

For those with violet eyes, choose flattering shades of taupe, olive, mauve or dark green.

Colour choices for blue eyes

Natural shades that tone with blue eyes are lilac, lavender, grey, silver, graphite, cool brown, taupe and soft violet. You can make your eyes appear even bluer with contrasting shades of terracotta, yellow gold, warm brown, russet, peach, copper or bronze.

Blue grey eyes look bluer with contrasting colours of golden brown, grey brown, grey, dusky rose, grey pink and blue green. And slate blue eye shadow is fabulous if your hair is grey.

Try bolder colours to make sure your eyes are the focal point of your face, but blend them well for a subtle effect.

BASIC RULES FOR EYE COLOUR

- Use dark colours in the crease below the brow bone to create depth and recess the eye.
- Use lighter colours on the lid area (particularly in the centre) to open up the eye.
- Use dark colours on the lid area to make the eye seem smaller.
- Always take colour from the outside corner, inwards and up, and blend, blend, blend.

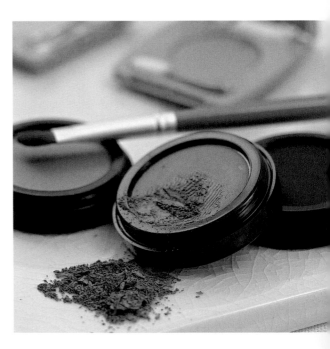

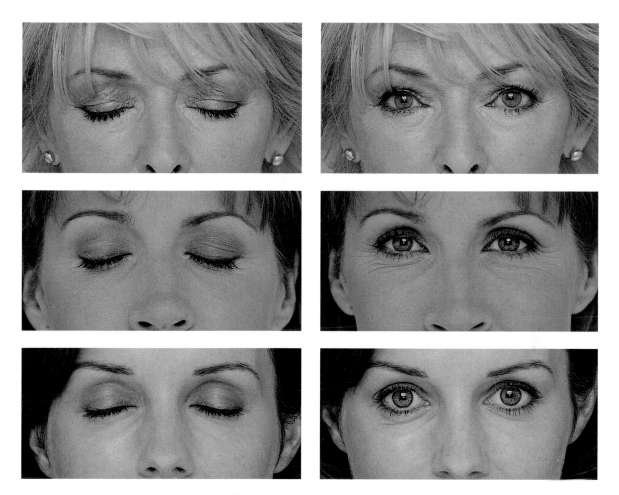

The same colour eyes can look dramatically different, depending on which eye shadow colour you choose.

Colour choices for brown eyes

Brown eyes can take most colours well, but consider your complexion when selecting your eye shadow colour – you don't want to make your eyes look too heavy. All the warm tones of brown, gold, tan, rust and bronze are good and natural looking for those with brown eyes. You can make brown eyes more beautiful with a stronger look using gold green, smoky forest green, soft brown, violet, cream or golden peach eye shadows.

Colour choices for green eyes

Green eyes are unusual and can vary greatly – from hazel green to blue green – so if you have green eyes you need to look closely at the coloured flecks in your iris to make your choices.

Natural colours to complement green are gold, soft green, cappuccino, cream and sand. Brownish apricot, bronze and warm browns always flatter green eyes, and so are a safe bet. For a dramatic look, emphasize your eyes' greenness by contrasting them with deep plum, violet, rose pink or flamingo.

EYEBROW MAGIC

- Start your eyebrow line directly above the inside corner of your eye and finish just slightly past the outside corner.
- Tweeze out hairs growing towards the centre of your nose and any other stragglers.
- Fill in any blanks with eyebrow pencil, using light, feathery strokes.
- Fix their shape by brushing colourless mascara through them.

LUSCIOUS LIPS

Lips are one area of the face that can give away your true age. Drooping corners and feathered lipstick will reveal your years unless, that is, you know the secrets to beautiful lips, with well-defined outlines and moist, perfectly coloured centres.

Some women wear the same colour lipstick they've always worn, but unfortunately lips, like complexions, change with age. Sharp outlines soften, skin becomes dry and colours turn bluer. Beautiful, full 'Cupid bows' disappear and corners droop, as your facial muscles relax. Fine lines appear running down from nose to mouth (most noticeably on smokers, who screw up their faces dragging on cigarettes). Lipstick also 'feathers' as you age, and this softening of edges is exaggerated if you use lipgloss instead of lipstick.

The challenge for mature women, therefore, is to overcome the effects of ageing and produce the best possible result. And it is still possible to have beautiful lips, with a bit of tender loving care.

TOP TIPS FOR LIPS

- To give lips the illusion of fullness, first outline them with a light-reflecting concealer, then follow with a nude lip liner, plus a natural-coloured lipstick.
- To counteract thin lips, choose lighter shades of lipstick (dark shades makes lips look mean). Also, dab a small amount of lipgloss on the centre of the lower lip, or, for a fresh-faced look, use lipgloss only on bare lips.
- To even out poorly defined lips, create a lip line that goes along the outermost border of the thinnest part and the innermost border of the thickest part. Using a slightly lighter lip colour on the smallest part also helps to make it look larger.
- To even out uneven-sized lips, dab some highlighter in the centre of the smaller lip – this will make it appear fuller.

Wands of colour

The range of lipstick colours available is extensive, from the palest pearly pink to the most vampish red, and from the most striking plum to a gothic black. With such a wide range to choose from it makes sense to have fun and experiment. Then, when you find a favourite, buy several and keep them in the fridge for future use.

To help lipstick stay in place all day, blot your lips with a tissue after the first coat, apply another coat, then lightly powder your lips with transparent powder to lock the colour in place. When your lipstick bullet seems empty, use a lip brush to dig out the remaining colour: you'll find another ten applications at least!

If you can't find the colour lipstick you want but you like the texture of a particular product, try mixing several colours with a lip brush until you get what you want. It's a great way of using up old lipsticks. If a lipstick is not the texture you like, add a little petroleum jelly – this is especially beneficial if your lips tend to be dry.

Colour choices

Many women find it difficult to decide which lipsticks suit them. Skin types and our individual chemical make-up vary dramatically. Many of you will know products that change colour on you over a period of time. If your lipstick does change colour, such as going dark or purple, it may be due to the acid content of your skin. So, choose a lipstick that doesn't have blue undertones or try applying a colourless barrier lipstick first, before the lip colour. If you want very pale colours, try lip balms, which also protect against sun and wind, or lipgloss, which contains less colour pigment but more clear balm.

LINING AND FILLING LIPS

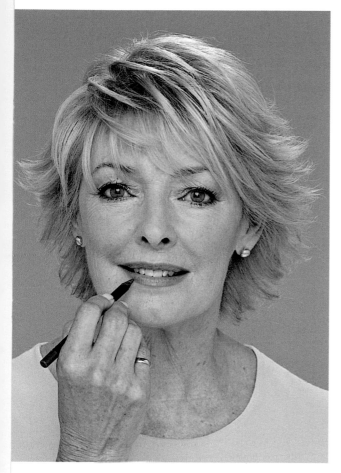

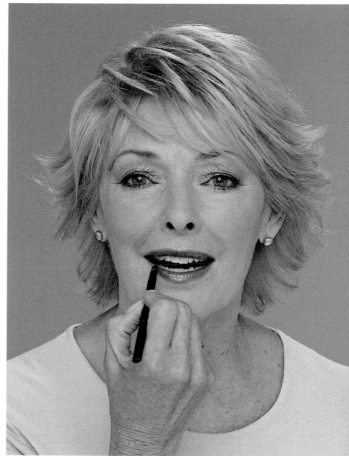

1 To sharpen your lip line, outline lips and avoid feathering, use a proper lip pencil. Keep it sharpened, but soften the tip with your finger. To create the effect of fuller lips, choose a lip liner in a shade that matches your natural lip colour, avoiding brown or coffee colours, which look too dated. Follow your natural lip line, being generous rather than going inside it, and try to even up the outline. Work from the outside corners of your top lip, drawing upwards to establish a good line. Lip liner has more colour pigment and stain than soft lipstick, which comes off easily by comparison. It is therefore a good idea to pencil a few light strokes of lip liner colour on to the lips themselves, which ensures that some colour and shape remain throughout the day.

2 Next fill in your lips with a lipstick colour close to your natural shade, using a lip brush to ensure even application. Lipsticks come in a huge variety, from strong pigments to soft, tinted lipgloss containing moisturizer. Remember, the darker your lipstick colour, the neater your outline must be, but dark colours can make mouths look pinched.

SUN PROTECTION FOR LIPS

Although the lips cannot produce melanin and tan, they can easily burn when exposed to the sun's harmful ultraviolet rays. The lower lip is a common area for skin cancer, so protect your lips and always wear a lip balm containing a minimum of SPF15 in winter or summer. Note that lip balms also protect your lips from the drying effects of sun and wind.

WHY FACIAL EXERCISE WORKS

The human face is the only part of the body where the muscles are attached directly to the skin instead of the bones. This unique arrangement means that by exercising the facial muscles, you can quickly affect the skin's tone and, ultimately, the shape of your face.

People express their emotions constantly, often without actually realizing it, and many of our facial movements become habitual as we respond to people or certain situations. We laugh at a friend's joke, smile when we meet loved ones or purse our lips in frustration when dealing with things we dislike. The emotions we experience and our reactions to them, in the form of our facial expressions, give each of us our individual look.

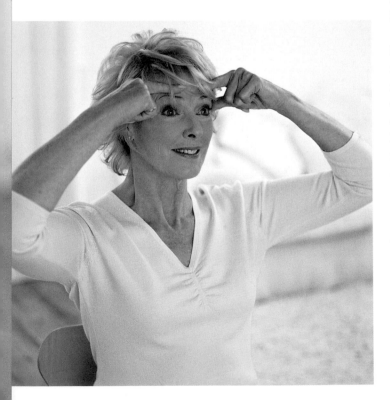

Combat ageing the natural way

There are many tempting solutions on offer to iron out wrinkles, lift up under-eye bags and plump out creases that involve operations and preparations. But they are expensive and not for the faint hearted. They are also not desirable for those of us who seek a more natural solution to looking younger. Facial exercise works in two ways: it helps to keep the muscles strong and fit, and allows the connective tissue around them to stay supple and relaxed. A mobile face always looks younger.

The exercises concentrate on individual muscles in key areas: the neck, mouth, cheeks, eyes and forehead. They isolate, work and tone the muscles repeatedly. Some exercises begin by concentrating on one side of the face and then repeating the movement on the other side. You will probably be surprised at how unevenly your facial muscles work from habit – most people find one side of their face easier to control than the other. Exercise also improves the adjoining connective tissue, increasing the supply of oxygen and nutrients to it. Furthermore, it stimulates cell growth in the elastic fibres within the collagen, which atrophy with age. But don't be afraid that you'll encourage wrinkles just because you are moving and contorting your face. Healthy, toned and supple skin will discourage the formation of lines when the strong underlying muscles work and relax back.

By practising simple eye exercises, you can brighten your eyes, reduce wrinkles and generally tighten the skin in the eye area, making your eyes look younger and less tired.

THE 'UPSIDE-DOWN' TEST

If you want a quick way of seeing the difference facial exercise could make to your face, then try this quick 'test', which will highlight your weak points. Hold a mirror in your hands, then bend over so that you are looking directly at your toes. Now look in the mirror. Your upside-down face will clearly show up any loose folds of skin. For some of us, it's not necessarily a pretty sight. But help is at hand, because these signs of the ageing process can be slowed down with facial exercises.

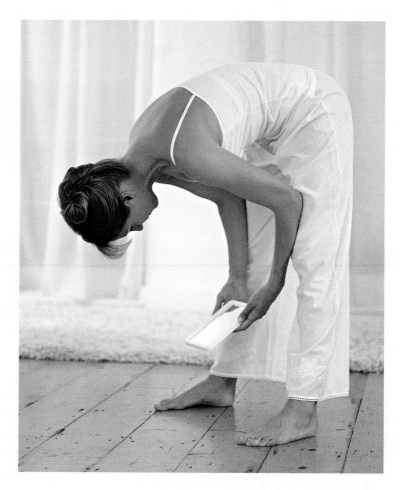

Any time, anywhere

Facial exercises can help to soften wrinkles, improve complexion and bring a sparkle to your eyes. They can be done at any time and in the comfort and privacy of your own home. No studio or equipment is required – just a chair to sit on and a mirror to look at – and you don't even need to wear a leotard. You can even do some of the exercises while driving in your car, travelling on a plane, walking the dog or watching television.

Practice makes perfect, and you need to perform the exercises correctly for them to have the desired effect, so try to remember the routine by using the quick reference guide at the end of the book (see pages 124–125).

Too many wrinkles and frowns are the result of stored up tension and stress – so learn to eliminate the tension through movement. You may find that doing the facial exercises will help you to de-stress, even more so while listening to music. Choose some slow, relaxing music, which will allow you to perform the movements with rhythm and control – and, what's more, will make the whole workout more enjoyable.

The younger you are when you start doing these facial gymnastics, the longer you will postpone the inevitable wrinkles: younger muscles are more elastic and build up bulk more quickly. Any improvement in the facial muscles will have a directly beneficial effect on facial skin tone. But, whatever your age, the experience can be more pleasurable if you finish it with a luxurious facial massage (see pages 96–97), ideally performed while keeping your eyes closed throughout. When you finally master the routine, allow yourself ample time to do it thoroughly and pamper yourself. You will find it's the most amazingly relaxing experience.

2 Stretch Out

This wonderful stretching exercise will have you holding your head high and feeling serene. And, at the same time, it will rid you of tension in your neck and upper back and increase the realm of mobility in this area, too.

The Stretch Out exercise works on the scalenus medius and sternocleidomastoideus muscles of the neck and shoulders (see pages 50–51). Stretching these muscles can help to release tension in your neck and upper back area.

The area on either side of your neck will be tight when you first start to exercise. With practice and regular stretching, however, your neck and upper back will become less stiff and soon allow more freedom of movement.

CAUTION!

If you suffer from neck problems, try doing this exercise while lying on a bed or the floor, and using a small pillow for support. Make sure that you tilt your head, as directed, only as far as is comfortable for you.

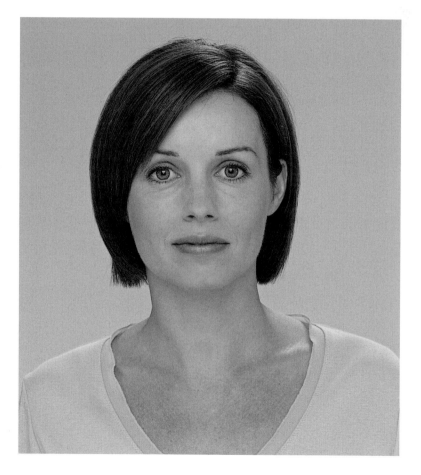

1 Keep your shoulders relaxed and down with chin parallel to the floor and look straight ahead. Breathe in.

'Stretching the scalenus medius and sternocleidomastoideus muscles can help to release tension in your neck and upper back area.'

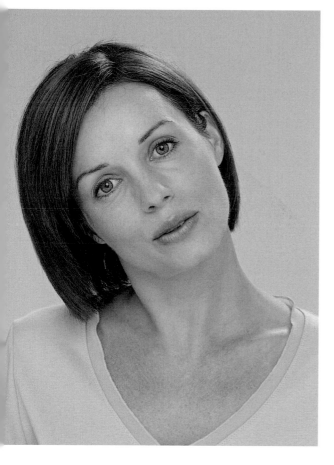

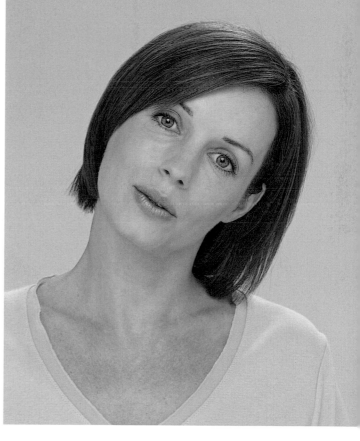

2 As you breathe out, bend your neck and take your right ear down towards your right shoulder, going just as far as is comfortable. Don't lift your shoulders up. Hold for 5 seconds and feel the stretch in the left side of your neck. Breathe in, bring your head back up to the centre and relax. Don't drop your head forwards or backwards.

3 Breathe out and repeat on the left side, taking your left ear towards your left shoulder. Hold for 5 seconds and feel the stretch in the right side of your neck, remembering to keep your shoulders down and relaxed. Breathe in once more, return to the centre and relax.

4 The Swan

Rediscover your elegant neck with this, the first of three throat exercises. With regular practice, it will firm up droopy jowls and tighten any sagginess in the throat, as well as releasing any pent-up tension in the throat and neck.

The Swan concentrates on the four main neck muscles: the sternocleidomastoideus, the scalenus medius, the omhyoideus and the sternohyoideus (see pages 50–51). As well as releasing tension and firming up the throat, it also lifts the breast tissue.

The Swan is also the position you will need to adopt for the next two exercises – The Goldfish (pages 62–63) and The Pelican (pages 64–65) – which also concentrate on firming up the jowls.

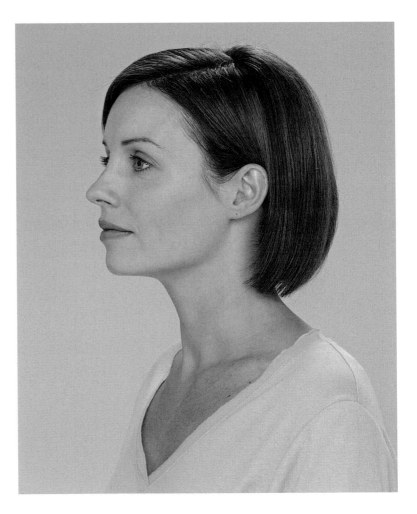

CAUTION!

If you suffer from neck problems, try doing this exercise while lying on a bed or the floor, and using a small pillow for support. If you suffer from a neck or upper back problem, do not take your head too far back.

1 Sit comfortably, remember your posture, keep your shoulders relaxed and down and look straight ahead. Breathe in.

'As well as releasing tension and firming up the throat, The Swan also lifts the breast tissue.'

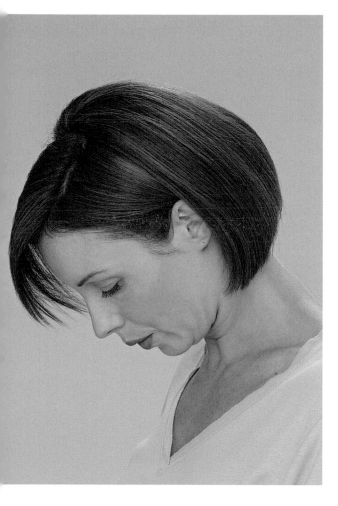
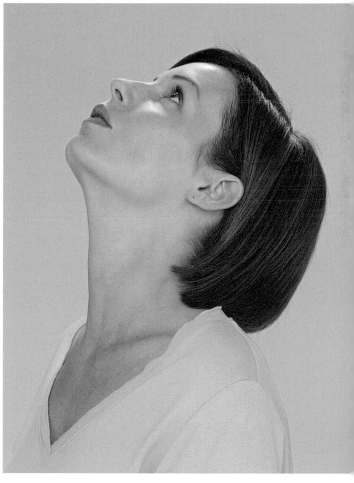

2 As you breathe out, drop your head forwards and pull your chin in to your chest. Hold for 5 seconds to release any tension felt in the back of your neck and head.

3 Now breathe in while carefully lifting your head, tipping it backwards (as far as is comfortable for you) and sticking out your chin. Keep your mouth closed. As you breathe out, lengthen your neck and feel the stretch under your chin. Hold for 5 seconds.

5 The Goldfish

If you've discovered that recently your jaw line is not what it used to be, or that a double chin is appearing on the horizon, practise The Goldfish. This stretching exercise will redefine your jaw line and tighten any slack in the throat area.

The Goldfish works on the sternohyoideus, digastricus and mentalis muscles of the chest, throat and under the chin (see pages 50–51). By stimulating these muscles to contract and relax, this stretch improves your jaw line and lifts saggy jowls. The exercise will also lift breast tissue and increase circulation to the face. Tipping the head backwards has the effect of making the muscles work even harder – with dramatic results.

CAUTION!

If you suffer from neck problems, try doing this exercise only as far as step 2. If you suffer from a neck or upper back problem but want to try step 3, do not take your head too far back.

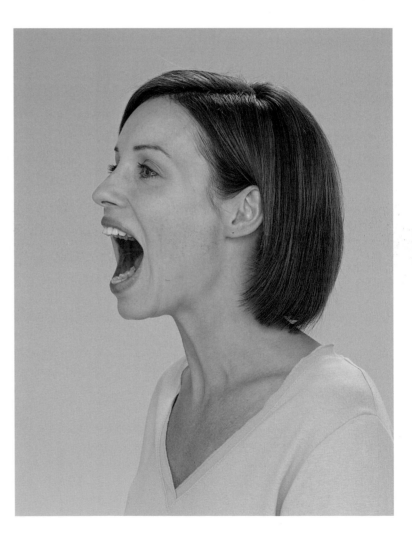

1 Keep your shoulders relaxed and down, and look straight at your mirror to learn this exercise before tipping your head back (see step 3). Breathe in and open your mouth as wide as possible.

'The Goldfish improves your jaw line and lifts saggy jowls.'

ADDING EXTRA STRETCH

Both The Goldfish and The Pelican (see pages 64–65) have been extended from the basic positions (reached in step 2 of each exercise) to combine with The Swan for step 3. This extra stretch gives both exercises a higher intensity, and you will be able to feel your neck, throat and chin working overtime as you tilt your head back. If your neck is stiff, stop at step 2 each time, until you feel ready to try step 3.

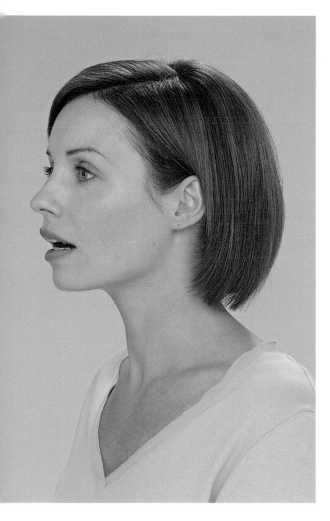

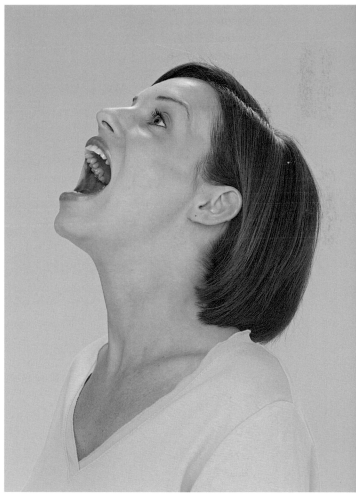

2 Breathe out through your nose as you close your lips together with a 'glugging' movement. Continue glugging like a goldfish several times until you become used to this rather strange movement.

3 Tilt your head backwards into The Swan position (see page 61). Stick your chin out, and repeat steps 1–2, pulling up your lower jaw hard each time you breathe out. Repeat 10 times, then relax.

6 The Pelican

As we grow older, the muscles of the jowl area, chin and neck lose tone and begin to sag; they are the first to show signs of age. Practise this exercise and wave that double chin goodbye, and watch as your jaw line is redefined, jowls banished and your saggy neck firmed up.

The Pelican works on the sternohyoideus, mentalis and digastricus muscles in the breastbone area, chin and lower jaw (see pages 50–51). To maintain a beautiful neck and firm jaw line, be sure to include the neck and jowl area in your regular skin-care routine as well as performing your facial exercises.

Double (or even triple) chins can result from excess weight; conversely, weight loss can cause slackness around the jowls. The Pelican is a strong movement that works the muscles under the chin and around the jaw and throat extremely hard. It is an excellent exercise with amazing results.

CAUTION!

If you suffer from neck problems, try doing this exercise only as far as step 2. If you suffer from a neck or upper back problem but want to try step 3, do not take your head too far back.

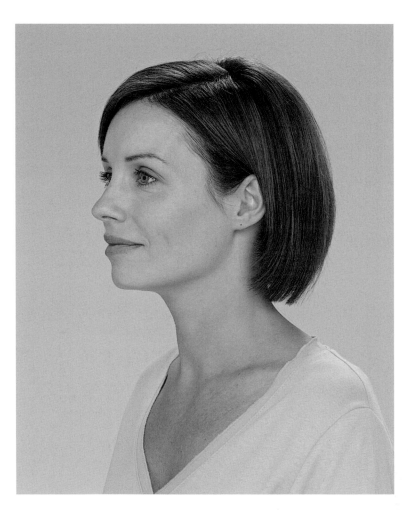

1 Keep your shoulders relaxed and down, and look straight ahead into your mirror to learn this exercise before extending the stretch by tipping your head back (see step 3). Breathe in.

'The Pelican will firm up your jaw line, smooth out your neck line and melt away a double chin.'

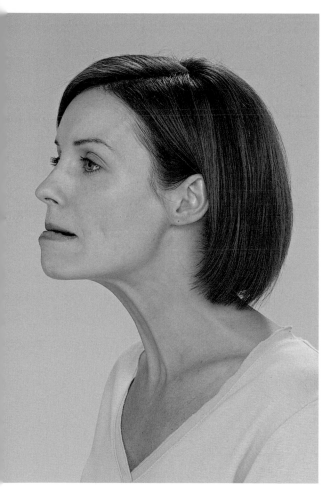

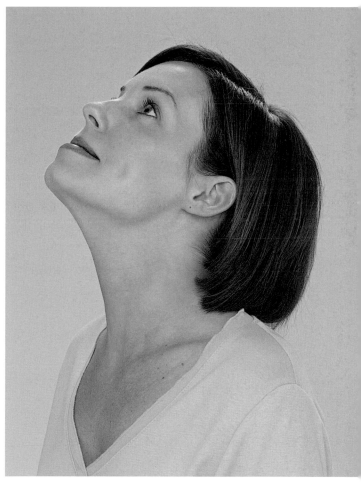

2 Breathe out and stick out your chin, pushing your lower jaw and teeth forwards as far as possible, and carefully try to bite your top lip softly. Hold for a count of 5 and feel the neck muscles working.

3 Tilt your head back into The Swan position (see page 61) and feel the stretch. Repeat steps 1–2 10 times, working the chin, jaw and neck muscles. Finally, relax with your head in an upright position.

7 The Lion

Roar like a Lion to release pent-up tension. This exercise boosts lymphatic drainage and the circulation, and promotes oxygenation of your skin and muscles. Discover the calm after the roar and find your hidden strength as you learn to feel good and look even better.

The Lion will boost your blood flow and create a general feeling of wellbeing. This unique and powerful exercise works on facial muscles, including those around the mouth, eyes, throat and cheeks, and on many others around your body. It assists the work of the previous jowl exercises (see pages 60–65) to prevent a double chin.

This exercise will de-stress and refresh you, and allow you to let go of pent-up tensions and emotions. You could do The Lion when you are in need of an instant energy boost, or in the car as an antidote to road rage.

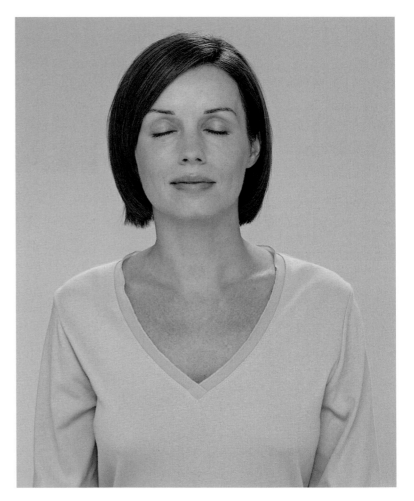

1 Keep your shoulders relaxed and sit upright with your head erect, hands relaxed on your thighs with fingers facing forward. Close your eyes and inhale deeply.

'The Lion will de-stress and refresh you, and allow you to let go of pent-up tensions and emotions.'

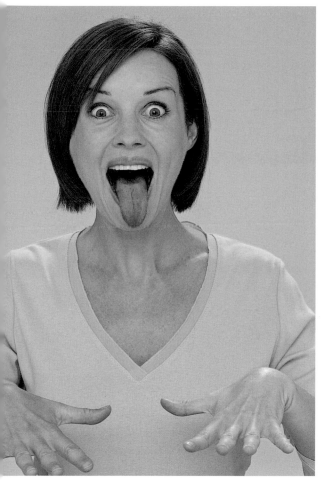

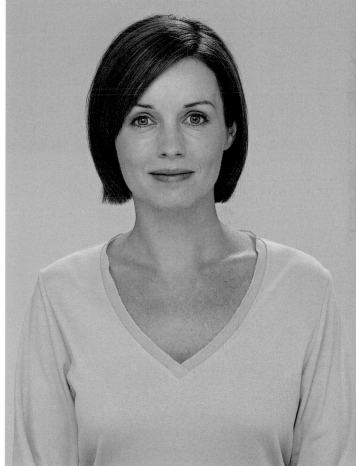

2 As you breathe out, open your eyes wide, stick out your tongue as far as possible (touch the tip to your chin if you can), lift your hands and forcibly spread out your fingers. Then, still on the same out-breath, roar like a fierce lion, as loud as you dare.

3 Enjoy the rush of adrenalin and feeling of release. Replace your hands on your thighs, relax your body and mind and relish a moment of peace and calm. If you like, repeat this uplifting experience once more.

8 Do As I Say

Longing for luscious lips? Work the muscles around your mouth with these simple sounds and say 'hello' to well-defined lips for good. This is also an excellent exercise for de-stressing and can be done any time, anywhere.

Do As I Say works major muscles around the mouth, including the orbicularis oris and triangularis muscles (see pages 50–51). The exercise releases tension around the mouth and tightness stored in the jaw and neck. It's an excellent de-stressing exercise – and you can do it while watching TV or travelling in the car.

The skin on our lips is drier than the rest of the face and is one of the first areas to show signs of ageing. Lips lose their shape and definition and can become thin and mean looking. Give them a boost, release tension and encourage circulation with this simple combination of three sounds.

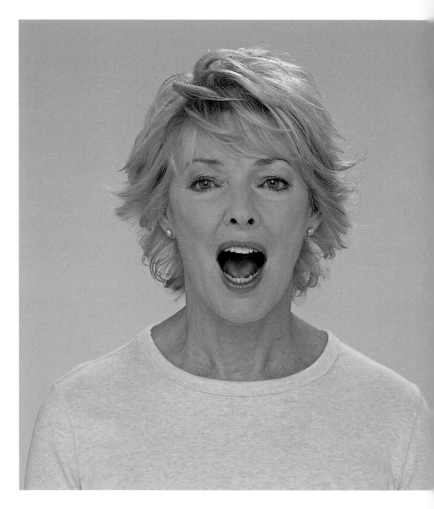

1 Keep your shoulders down and relaxed. Broaden out your back and look straight ahead. Breathe out as you simply open your mouth (drop your lower jaw down to your chin) and make the noise 'uh'. Then, close your mouth and breathe in.

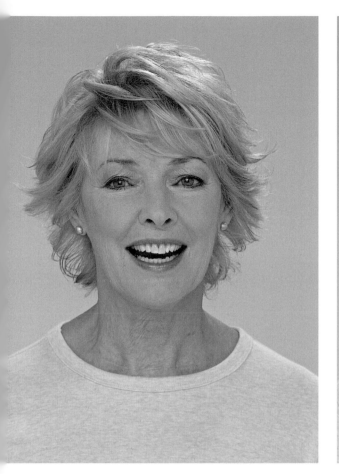

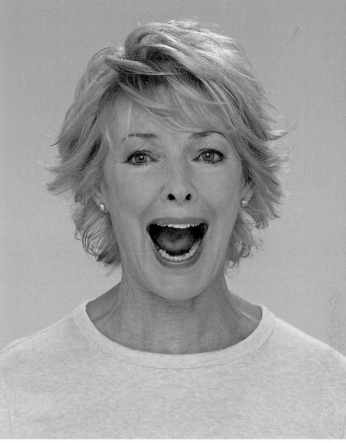

2 Open your mouth, part your lips, pull the corners back sideways over your teeth, as wide as possible and, as you breathe out, make the noise 'ee'. Notice your cheek and neck muscles working, too. Close your mouth and breathe in.

3 Open your mouth very wide this time, drop your lower jaw down as far as possible and pull the corners out as far as you can. With this big mouth, breathe out, making the sound 'ah'. Then close your mouth. All three sounds form the exercise and are performed one after the other, in sequence. Repeat 'uh', 'ee' and 'ah' 10 times.

'Do As I Say is an excellent de-stressing exercise – and you can do it while watching TV or travelling in the car.'

9 Whistlestop

As we age, the muscles around the mouth can lose their tone and become saggy. This exercise will banish droopy mouths and nearby sagging muscles – and you can whistle whatever tune you like.

Whistlestop works on the triangularis, orbicularis oris and buccinator muscles around the lips and cheeks in particular (see pages 50–51). The exercise will help to lift the corners of the mouth, which droop when we show our displeasure and sag as the muscles around our mouths lose their tone as we get older. Whistlestop can also help to lessen the appearance of unsightly vertical lines running down from the nose to the upper lip, which appear with age.

Stand in front of a mirror and purse your lips and try whistling. Watch what happens around your mouth. You will see an accumulation of vertical lines forming – a sure sign of ageing, and one that is emphasized if you are a smoker.

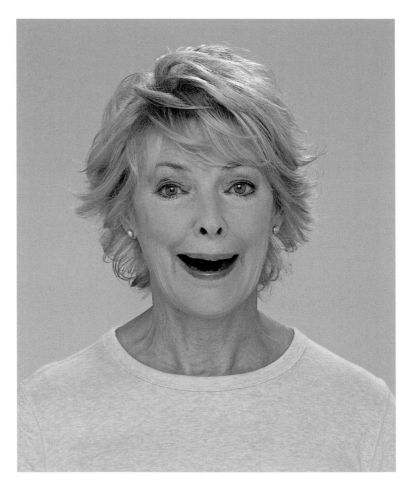

1 Keep your shoulders down and relaxed and remember to sit up straight. Breathe in and stretch out your top lip and pull it taut over your top teeth. Locate the muscles at the corner of your mouth, pull them up and feel your cheek muscles working as you breathe out.

'Whistlestop will help to lift the corners of the mouth, which sag as the muscles around our mouths lose their tone as we get older.'

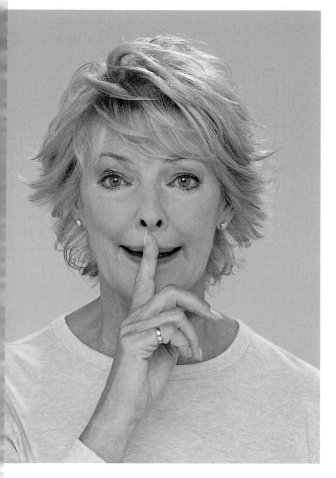

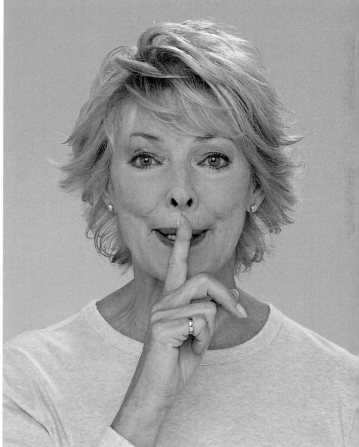

2 Place your index finger in the middle of your upper lip (keeping it taut) and breathe in. Now you are in the correct position to whistle without forming horrid vertical lines.

3 Pull up the corners of your mouth hard, bring your bottom jaw up and forwards. With lower teeth showing, whistle through your teeth as you breathe out for a count of 5. Make as much noise as you can while keeping your upper lip stretched over your teeth. Do not purse your lips. Repeat steps 1–3 10 times.

11 The Snarl

Learn to control the symmetry of your face in this exercise, where you snarl like a dog. The Snarl will lift and tone your cheek muscles, help to keep your face mobile and result in more even and alert expressions.

If you have to describe a person, place or object that you dislike, you may already be doing part of this exercise unconsciously with a snarl on one side of your nose. This exercise uses the quadratus labii superioris (which works the upper lip muscle) as well as the zygomaticus (cheekbone muscle), which creates a smile (see pages 50–51). Many people use one side of their face more than the other – and you may well find that this is true for you during the following movements.

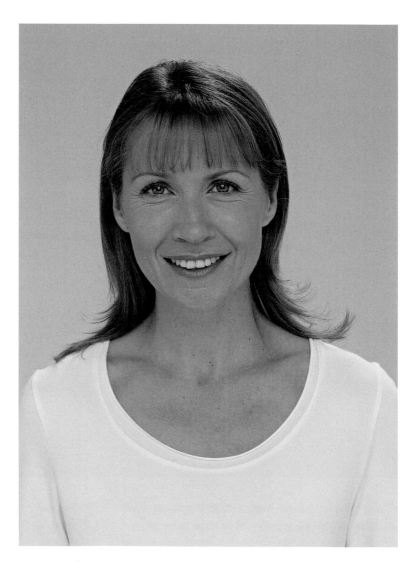

1 Keep your shoulders relaxed and down and look straight ahead into the mirror.

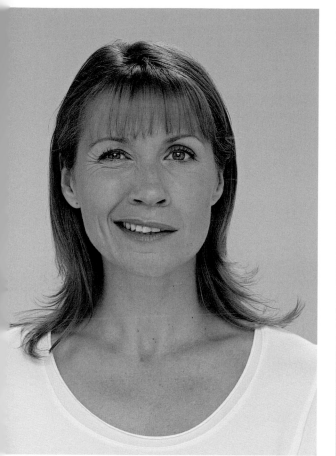

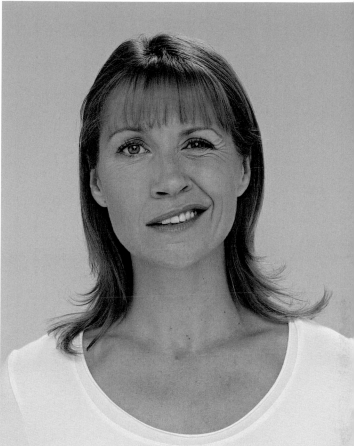

2 Keep your lips relaxed and, as you breathe in, pull a snarl on the right side of your face only. You'll need to pull up your lip, nostril and cheek towards your right eye as hard as you can for a count of 5. Let your face relax with a slow, controlled movement, again for a count of 5, as you breathe out. Repeat the exercise 5 times on the right side.

3 Continue this exercise, repeating it on your left side. Breathe in, then snarl up your left nostril, lip and cheek 5 times, controlling both the up and down movements. The facial muscles work hard and will quiver. You may find it more difficult to control one side than the other, but with practice you'll soon be expert at snarling on both sides of your face.

'Many people use one side of their face more than the other – and you may well find that this is true for you during The Snarl.'

12 The Cheshire Cat

Give yourself something to smile about: this exercise will tone up facial muscles, improve facial mobility and re-define the contours of your face. Plus, it can help to make your facial features and movements more symmetrical.

Like The Snarl, The Cheshire Cat exercise locates, concentrates on and works individual muscles alternately on either side of the face. The exercise works four different muscles: the quadratus labii superioris, the zygomaticus, the orbicularis oris and the buccinator (see pages 50–51). Regular practice will help your facial features to appear more symmetrical by toning up muscles and improving facial mobility on both sides of the face. What's more, it will lift the cheek area, re-define the contours of the face and help to equalize your facial movements. It's worth spending the time to locate the muscles and then concentrate on working them independently on either side of the face.

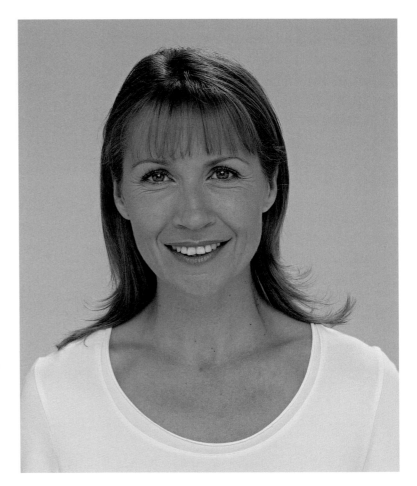

1 Keep your shoulders relaxed and down and look straight ahead.

'The Cheshire Cat will lift the cheek area, re-define the contours of the face and help to equalize your facial movements.'

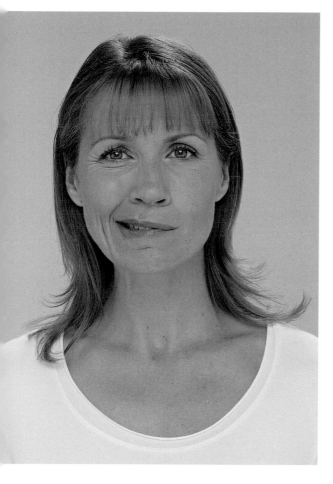

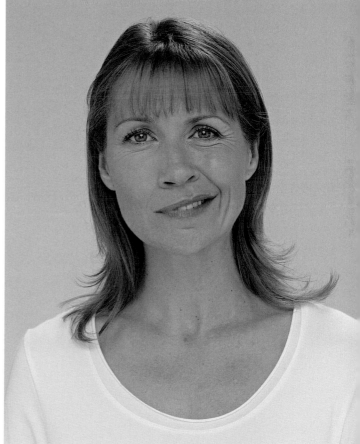

2 With teeth and lips together, breathe in, and at the same time make a slow half smile on the right side of your face only. Take the smile out as wide as you can towards your ear, working both the cheek and the lips. Breathe out and relax the smile to the centre. Repeat 5 times on the right.

3 Breathe in and this time take the half smile wide out to the left, and slowly back to the centre as you breathe out. Repeat 5 times. Concentrate on both the up and the down movements. Muscles do become easier to control with practice, so make facial exercises such as this a regular part of your workout.

13 The Cow

Plump up those cheeks and improve your complexion both at the same time with this simple exercise that will really get you chewing the cud. It's a strong exercise that works on the four muscles of the jaw and cheeks.

The Cow exercise works the masseter (the chewing muscle that closes the jaw), the temporalis (which enables the jaw to close), the zygomaticus and the orbicularis oris – both of which help to move the mouth in various directions (see pages 50–51).

This exercise will release tension in the jaw, mouth and cheek area. If you do this exercise properly, you will definitely feel that you have worked the muscles. As with the two previous exercises – The Snarl (see pages 74–75) and The Cheshire Cat (see pages 76–77) – The Cow must be performed first to one side of the face and then to the other.

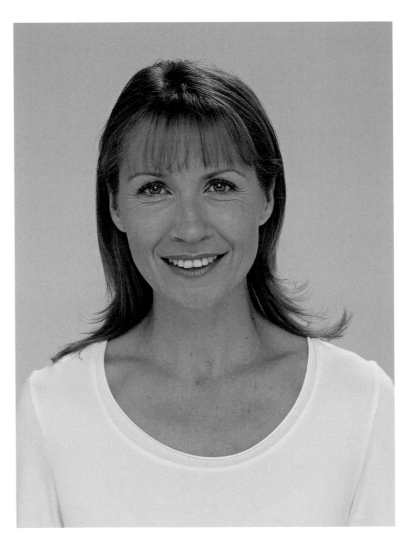

1 Keep your shoulders relaxed and down and look straight ahead into the mirror. Remember your posture and sit upright. Breathe in.

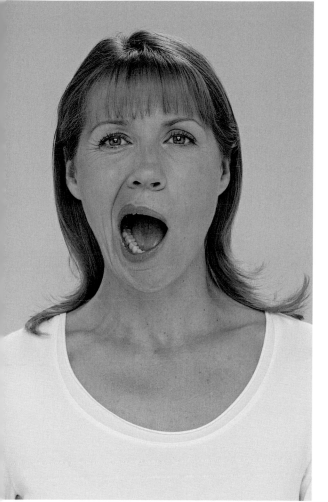
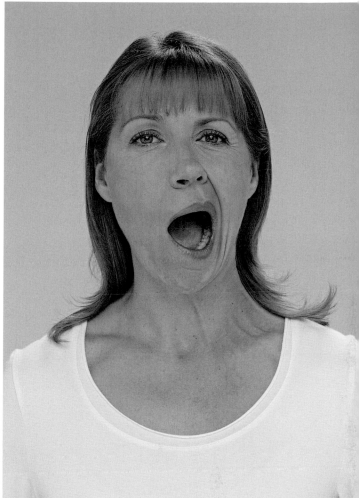

2 Open your mouth as wide as possible and, moving the right side of your face only, breathe out as you lift your right cheek up. Try taking your mouth out towards your right ear, and purposely work your right cheek in a circular movement. (It's a good idea to imagine you are chewing the cud or to try gently biting the inside of your cheek to get the action.) Keep your left cheek relaxed while you work the right cheek. Repeat 5 times.

3 Now, it's time to work the left cheek. Start with a relaxed position and breathe in. Open your mouth wide and as you breathe out work your left cheek hard, as you did the right one, with a slow, controlled movement; then repeat 5 times.

'The Cow will release tension in the jaw, mouth and cheek area.'

14 Blow Away

After all the effort of the workout so far, now is the time to give your face a rest with this simple facial relaxation technique. After this well-deserved bit of time out, you will be moving on to perform six exercises to improve your eyes.

For any exercise to be effective, you need to exert and work the muscle, then follow the exertion with a period of relaxation to give the muscle a chance to recover. The same principle of work and relaxation applies to our facial exercises, too.

We have been concentrating our efforts on many individual muscles throughout the facial workout, but now it's time to give them a chance to unwind before moving on to the eyes.

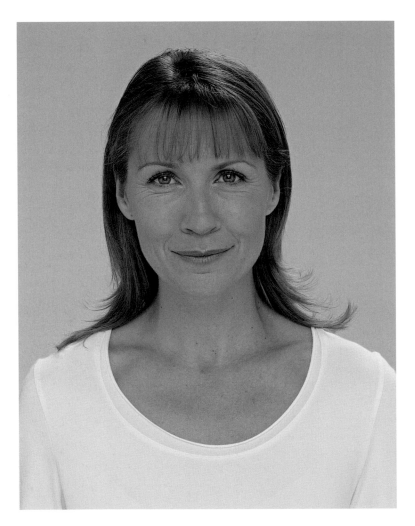

1 Keep your shoulders relaxed and down and look straight ahead. Take a deep breath in though your nose and keep your lips just softly together (don't purse them).

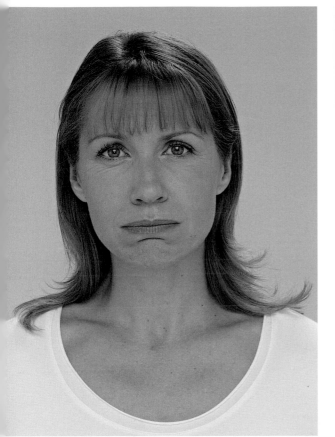

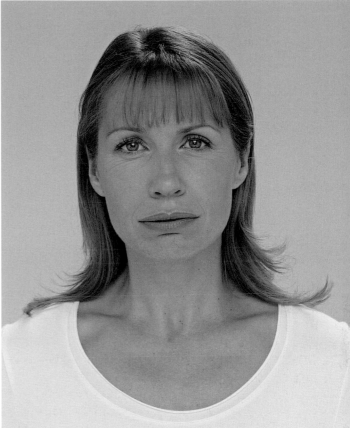

2 Blow as much of the air from your lungs as possible into your cheeks and lips. Fill them up and puff them out like balloons to relax them.

3 Keep your mouth very soft indeed and allow the air in your cheeks to escape slowly through your now slightly parted lips, for a count of 5. Let all the air out and relax your cheeks. Then breathe in and repeat 5 times.

'For any exercise to be effective, you need to exert and work the muscle, then follow the exertion with a period of relaxation to give the muscle a chance to recover.'

15 Bright Eyes

As we get older, our eyes still look youthful, even though the wrinkled skin surrounding them may tell a truer tale of our age. Use this relaxing eye exercise to maintain that young-looking sparkle in your eyes and let them shine.

Bright Eyes works by relaxing the ring muscle that circles the eye (the orbicularis oculi, see pages 50–51), which is responsible for many of the lines associated with laughter and smiling. This exercise also helps to relax the muscles of the eye itself. Modern life can wreak havoc on our eyes – during our work and our relaxation. Many of us stare for too long at our TV or computer screens, without taking the necessary break to prevent eyestrain. Ideally, for the health of your eyes, you should look away from concentrating on near objects (computer screens, books, TV screens) every 20 minutes or so to give your eyes the chance of focusing on objects further away in the distance. Whenever you feel stressed, Bright Eyes can help your eyes to feel refreshed in no time and can prevent tension headaches.

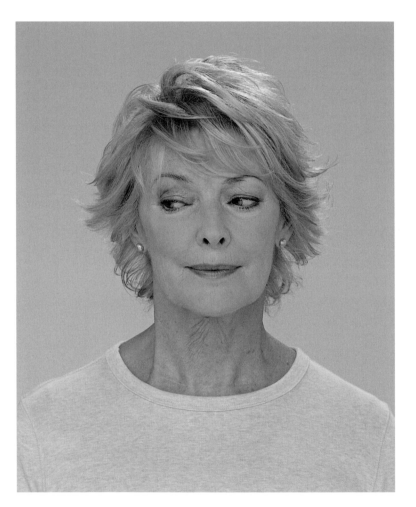

1 Keep your chin parallel with the floor and look straight ahead with shoulders facing the front. Now, breathe in. Keeping your head and shoulders completely still, look over to your right side, focus and breathe out.

'Whenever you feel stressed, this simple exercise can help your eyes to feel refreshed in no time and can prevent tension headaches.'

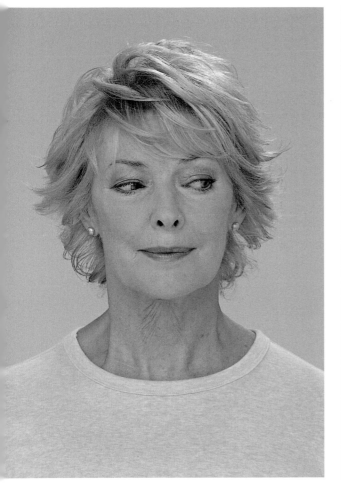

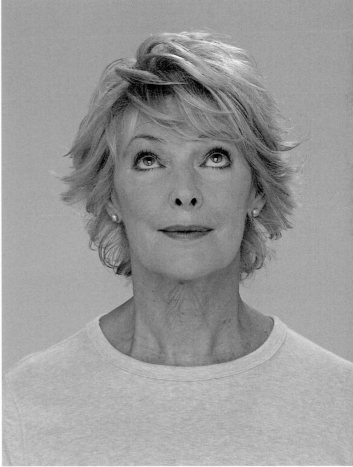

2 Breathe in, drop your eyes to look at your lap, focus and breathe out. Now breathe in and take eyes left, focus and breathe out. (Be sure to keep your head still throughout and your chin parallel with the floor: it's just your eyes doing the work.)

3 Breathe in, take eyes up to the ceiling, focus and breathe out. Bring them back to the centre and then off to repeat these movements on the right side. Controlling your eye movements carefully, repeat the cycle 5 times.

17 Downers

Lines under and around the eyes are a common feature of growing old, but fortunately there's a lot you can do to counter these wrinkles. This facial lifesaver can prove problematic to get the hang of, but once you have, you, and all your friends, will witness the fabulous results.

Lines under the eyes are signs of overtiredness, eyestrain or overindulgence in caffeine, alcohol or drugs. Strained eyes appear worse when accompanied by dark under-eye circles or bags.

Of all the facial exercises, Downers is the one that many people find tricky to conquer. If the exercise is done correctly there is only a small movement seen under the eye; so first you need to locate, observe and practise. Don't despair if you don't succeed first time, you will eventually and the results will be worthwhile. The exercise tones the orbicularis oculi ring muscle (see pages 50–51) and stimulates the circulation and lymphatic drainage system in the area. The small movement of Downers most closely resembles a cat narrowing its eyes.

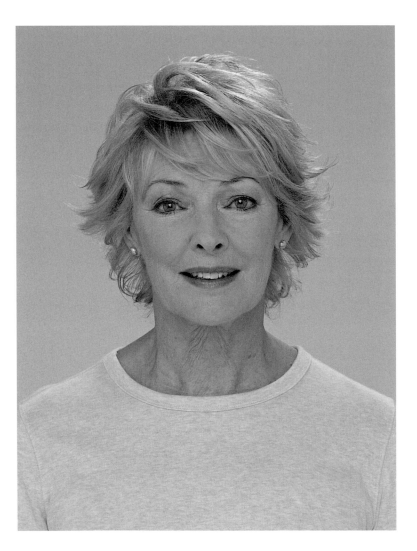

1 Keep your shoulders relaxed and down and look straight ahead at the mirror so that you can observe the small movement involved.

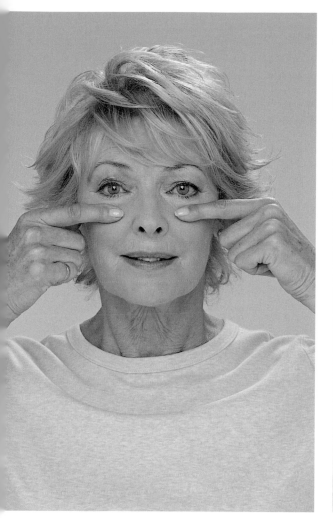

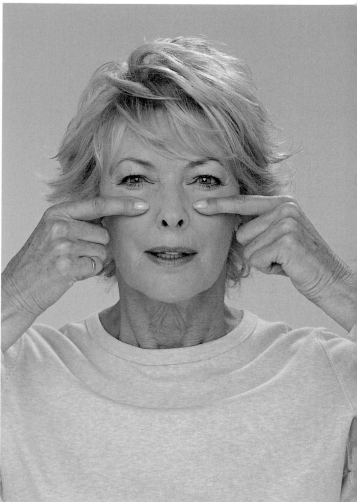

2 Place your forefingers horizontally under the centre of your eyes, and put your thumbs in front of your ears. Feel the top of your cheekbones, and hold the muscle and skin firmly in place to offer resistance. Take care not to drag or stretch the delicate skin under the eye. Breathe in.

3 As you breathe out, contract and squeeze up the tiny muscle under your lower eyelids. Don't screw up your eyes completely – just pull up the lower lids using the muscle under the eyes. (Be careful not to push up the skin and muscle with your fingers.) Hold for a count of 5, then repeat 10 times.

'The small movement of Downers most closely resembles a cat narrowing its eyes.'

18 Crow's Feet

Squinting gives us crow's feet. Whether we squint because of bright sun, tension or tiredness, the final effect is the same – lines at the outside corners of the eyes. Give wrinkles the heave-ho with this easy exercise to soften lines and relax those tired eyes.

As with Downers (see pages 86–87), Crow's Feet also exercises the ring of muscle around the eye, the orbicularis oculi (see pages 50–51). Poor eyesight, bright sunshine, tension, emotion and tiredness may cause us to squint badly. Squinting can become a habit and results in lines forming at the outside corners of the eye. Often referred to as crow's feet, these lines resemble a bird's claw.

This exercise can help to soften the lines and relax tension around the eyes. But, unlike Downers, you need to squint the entire eye, as if you were shielding your eyes from the sun's powerful rays. Once again, we use the forefingers to provide some resistance to the muscle's movement.

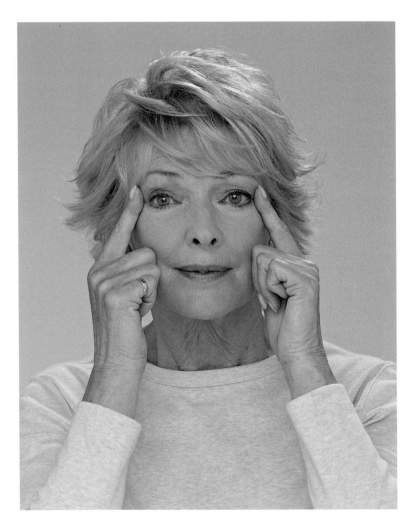

1 Keep your shoulders relaxed and down and look straight ahead. Place the pads of your forefingers horizontally on the skin and bone at the outside corners of your eyes.

'The Crow's Feet exercise can help to soften the lines and relax tension around the eyes.'

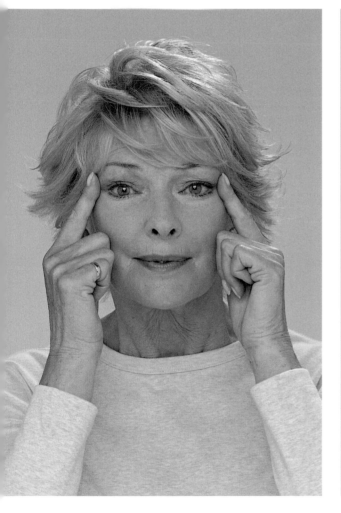

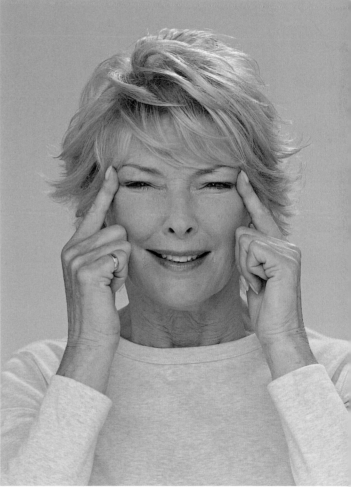

2 Pull back your fingers ever so slightly to create some resistance, but take care not to stretch the skin as you do so. Breathe in.

3 As you breathe out squint up the entire eye, pushing hard against the resistance, and hold for a count of 5. Feel the muscles at the sides of your eyes quivering and working. Repeat 10 times.

19 Cross Lines

As we get older, repeated frowning and other facial expressions push the fat in the skin into furrows. And as the amount of collagen and elastin declines with age, these furrows can become permanent. Use this exercise to prevent tell-tale signs of stress and to banish lines.

Cross Lines works and strengthens the frontalis muscles and the orbicularis oculi ring muscle (see pages 50–51). It will help to soften the vertical lines in the centre of your forehead and release tension.

Our emotions and facial habits are being continually etched upon our faces throughout life. If we laugh a lot, we create laughter lines around the eyes. But habitual frowning eventually creates a cross look, with two vertical lines forming between the eyebrows. Toning up the muscles can help to create a softer look, and the exercise may remind you not to frown.

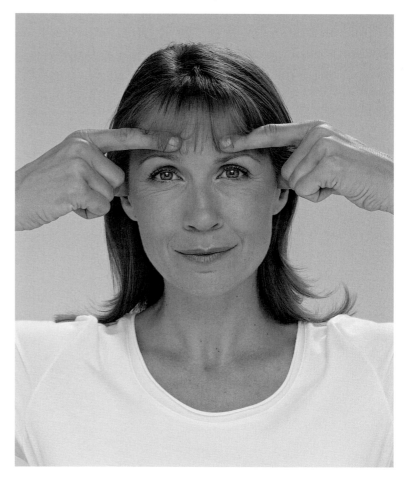

1 Keep your shoulders relaxed and down and look straight ahead. Place the pad of each forefinger above and towards the inner end of each eyebrow, with your thumbs in front of your ears.

'Use Cross Lines to reverse the effect of habitual frowning, which creates a cross look, with two vertical lines between the brows.'

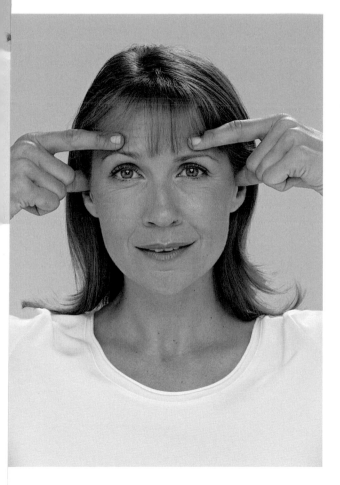

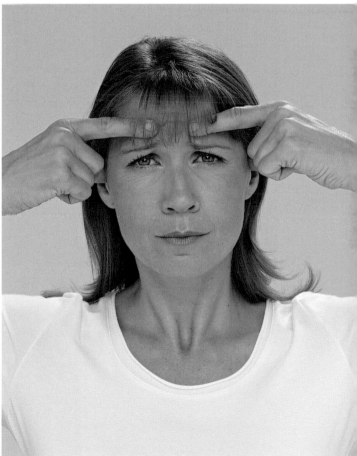

2 Use your fingers to press the skin and muscle firmly against your forehead bone. Now, pull your fingers slightly apart, easing out the vertical frown lines. Take care not to drag the skin unnecessarily. Breathe in.

3 As you breathe out, hold the lines apart, and, for a count of 5, try hard to create the frown in the centre of your forehead against the fingers' resistance. This will tone the muscles and lessen the lines. As you execute the movement, you will feel the muscles work and quiver. Relax and repeat 10 times.

IT'S TIME TO RELAX

What could be more luxurious and relaxing than to wind down at the end of the Fresh Face Workout with a facial massage – perhaps even using your favourite essential oils? Whatever your skin type, there is an oil that will be just perfect for your skin, leaving it supple and scented.

Massage stimulates both the blood and lymph circulations, which are slowed by poor sleep, lack of exercise, bad nutrition, shallow breathing and overexposure to pollutants. Blood vessels transport nutrients and oxygen around the body, while the lymphatic drainage system collects and carries away waste products – including toxins – from the areas being massaged. Aromatherapy massage using scented oils has wide-ranging benefits that vary depending on the essential oils you choose to use. The pressure applied during an aromatherapy massage increases the blood flow, and the oils' healing powers are absorbed by the skin and inhaled through the nose.

CAUTION!

Never use essential oils neat: they should always be diluted with a carrier oil. Whatever your skin type, always do a skin patch test first. Place a diluted drop of oil on the skin and leave for 24 hours. If there is any adverse reaction, don't use it.

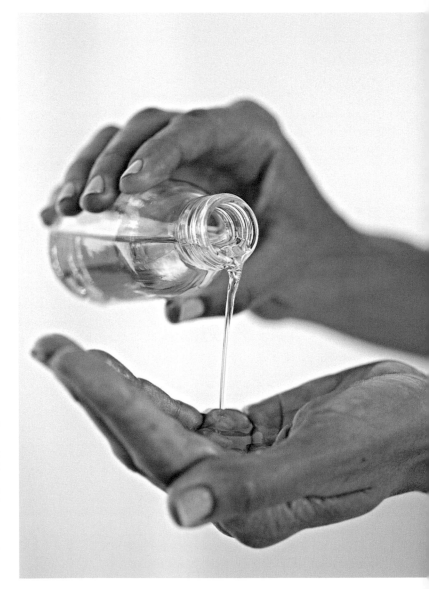

Blend your favourite essential oil with a carrier oil, then use to pamper your skin.

AVOID MINERAL OILS

Inexpensive mineral oils have a long shelf-life and rarely produce allergic reactions. However, they don't contain any beneficial nutrients and aren't readily absorbed by the skin; instead, these oils sit on the surface like a thin plastic film, blocking the skin's pores by 40–60 per cent. Mineral oils successfully stop moisture evaporating but deprive skin of vital oxygen, causing blackheads and blemishes. If used in the long term, these oils reduce the skin's ability to produce its own oil.

Which oils to choose

Your skin's natural oil levels diminish with age, and so oil from your diet is needed to top them up. Oil applied externally cannot replace it, but natural plant oils can benefit your skin's condition by reducing the escape of moisture. Pure vegetable oils are easily absorbed and both nourish and lubricate the skin. They also don't discourage your skin's own oil production or spread a suffocating film over your skin (as mineral oils do, see above).

Vegetable and nut oils provide a perfect lubricating oil for massaging, but oiling can overheat delicate, sensitive skins and cause pores to open too wide during massage, so choose your oils wisely. Oily skins already produce enough natural oil from their sebaceous glands for fingers to glide over without the need for extra oil, while some people feel that the delicate sensitivity of finger to face is lessened by using oil during massage.

Vegetable oils have one disadvantage: they go rancid, particularly when exposed to air. However, the addition of the antioxidant vitamin E can prevent this. Vegetable oils contain beneficial fatty acids and fat-soluble vitamins, which the skin slowly absorbs. When shopping for vegetable oils, choose cold-pressed versions from health food shops, as many commercial oils are hot-pressed, which that means all the nutrients have been destroyed.

Oils for your skin type

Which vegetable oil you should use depends on your skin type. Dry skin, for example, benefits from thick and sticky oils, rich in saturated fatty acids. Although these take longer to absorb, they are efficient at curbing water loss. A greasy skin, on the other hand, benefits from oils containing a high percentage of thinner polyunsaturated fats, which are absorbed quickly. All skin types benefit from borage and evening primrose oils, both of which possess special anti-ageing properties and are rich in gamma-linoleic acid (GLA). GLA strengthens skin cells, decreases moisture loss and helps destroy skin-ageing free radicals. But be aware that both these oils have a tendency to go rancid, so choose versions with added vitamin E to prevent this.

Your massage blend

Select your carrier or base oil (see below for one suited to your skin type) and add your favourite essential oil. Essential oils can be expensive and are powerful, so blend one part to seven parts of carrier oil. (When choosing your essential oil, check with a qualified aromatherapist if you are pregnant or breastfeeding, and inform your doctor in case there are any contraindications with ongoing medical treatment.)

TOP CARRIER OILS FOR DRY, AGEING SKIN

- Apricot
- Avocado
- Macadamia
- Wheatgerm

TOP CARRIER OILS FOR NORMAL SKIN

- Olive
- Almond
- Sunflower
- Sesame

TOP CARRIER OILS FOR OILY SKIN

- Hazelnut
- Peach kernel
- Thistle
- Hypericum

FIVE STEPS TO YOUTHFUL RADIANCE

Tension surfaces on your face as frown lines, but other tell-tale signs are rigid jaws, staring eyes and pursed lips. Smooth out frown lines and relax your face completely with this powerful pick-me-up: a facial massage in the privacy of your own home.

Facial massage is a wonderful way of releasing tension and reducing stress, leaving your face looking relaxed and younger. Light massage of your facial muscles stimulates the circulation and makes your complexion glow. To avoid damaging or stretching your skin, apply some moisturizer, your favourite aromatherapy blend or some vegetable oil to your forehead. Use only light, feathery touches – you are not trying to move the skin or muscle as you did in some of the exercises.

You'll need to practise this short, relaxing routine while looking into the mirror to start with. But once you've learnt the five steps, you'll benefit more if you perform the sequence with your eyes closed. You'll know from the feeling of your fingers on your skin if you're performing the steps correctly. Take your time, relax and enjoy the pampering sensation, and, hopefully, when you've finished, you will experience a feeling of calm and wellbeing.

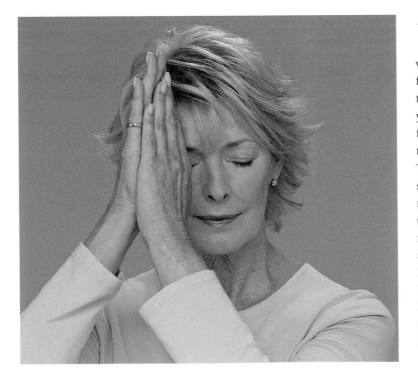

1 Sit in the correct posture (see page 52). Place your hands vertically on the centre of your forehead so that your forefingers touch the hairline. Gently slide your right fingers up and your left fingers down your forehead from the eyebrows up into the hairline. Then, reverse the brisk but delicate sawing movement, moving your right fingers down and your left up. Work your fingers out to your right temple, back to the centre and then repeat on the left side. Repeat these movements twice. Bring your hands down on to your lap, with your palms uppermost and your thumbs and middle fingers touching.

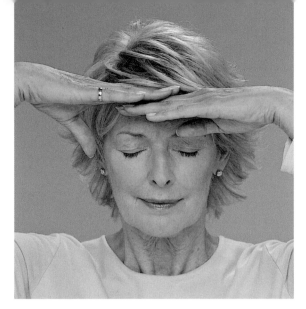

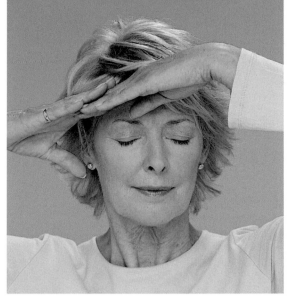

2 Breathe deeply and relax your neck and shoulders. Now, bring your hands up, with the palms facing downwards and your fingers horizontally on top of each other, and place them on the bridge of your nose. Slide your fingers backwards and forwards, gently working up over the nose and forehead into the hairline and back down again. Repeat twice.

3 Now, slant your hands and incline them to the right. With backwards and forwards movements, work diagonally over and up into the hairline at your right temple and back to the centre. Repeat twice, then do this 3 times on the left side. When you have finished, place your hands gently in your lap as before. Breathe deeply and relax your shoulders.

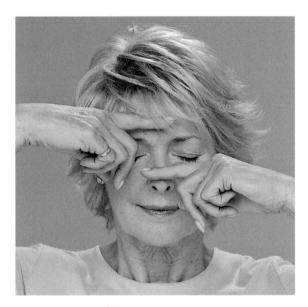

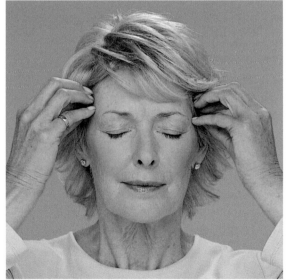

4 Bring your hands to your face and lightly place both forefingers horizontally on your nose. Use a light, feathery touch to stroke from the nose to the hairline with alternate forefingers, one after the other in a circular motion. Use delicate strokes, and move up over your nose, forehead and into your hairline 10 times to help you relax. Then rest your hands in your lap as before.

5 Finally, bring your hands up and place all your fingertips lightly at the centre of the forehead at the hairline. Trace the hairline out across your forehead, down the sides of your face and past your ears. Then sweep them round to your chin and then up over your nose and back to your forehead. Repeat this 5 times. Place your hands in your lap as before and breathe deeply, relax and enjoy a moment of tranquillity.

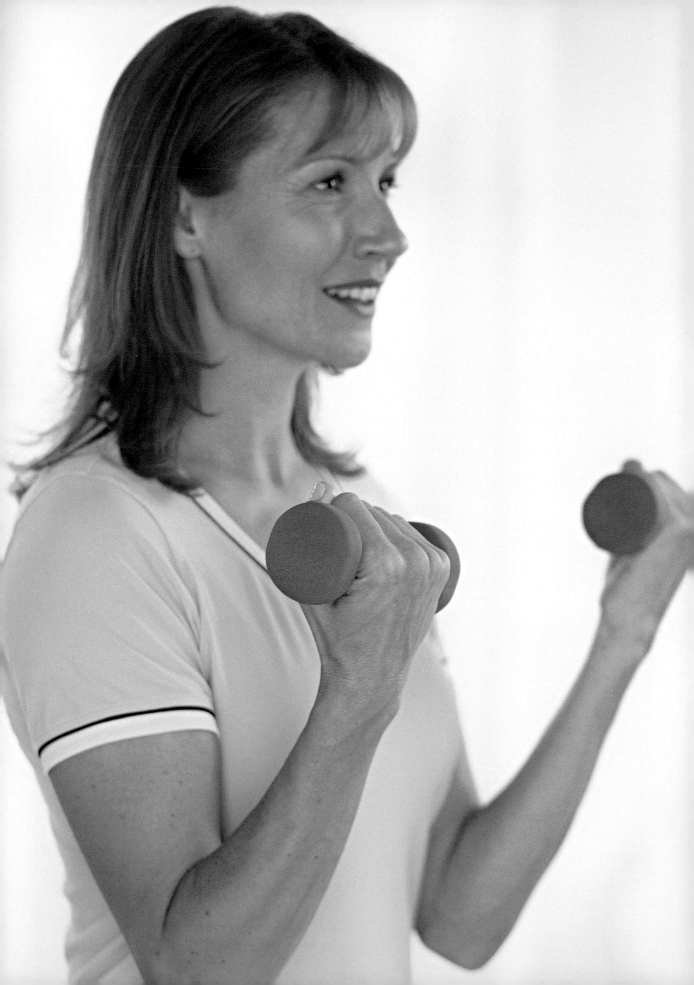

Stress-busting

Your skin is the outward and obvious sign that tells the world about your lifestyle. If you don't eat properly, don't get enough sleep or feel stressed, your skin is likely to suffer. By learning to recognize the signs of stress (and by avoiding stressful situations as much as possible), you can lessen the effect stress has on your face. What's more, having a positive attitude can work wonders for both your health and your wellbeing, and prepares you to beat the stress in your life.

STRESS AND AGEING

The accumulated pressures of everyday life – also known as stress – can work for or against you. Positive stress motivates you to feel in charge of events; negative stress makes you feel that events control you. Find out how stress affects your body and how it shows on your face.

Stressful events are not new and, as if to prove it, our bodies have a very primitive response to stress – known as the 'fight or flight' response. When our ancestors were faced with life-threatening situations, their bodies needed to be ready to face the danger or run away, depending on the situation. Most stressful situations today are not life-threatening, but the body still responds in the same way and switches to 'red alert' when faced with a highly stressful situation: hormones flood the bloodstream, the breathing rate increases, the heart pumps faster, the circulation diverts blood to the brain, muscles and lungs (and away from the skin), the blood pressure rises and the liver releases stores of sugar needed for that extra energy burst. You

may be familiar with how these biological actions make you feel – racing heart, shaking hands, dry mouth and butterflies in the stomach.

Many different types of event can be stressful – for example losing a partner, divorce, changing jobs or financial worries – and even happy occasions, such as weddings and the birth of a child, can load on the stress. But by having a calm approach and positive outlook you can increase your capacity to cope with stress, making it more of a positive factor in your life.

Positive and negative stress

We all need a level of positive stress to make our lives rewarding, whether it is a degree of competition or a challenge. Life would be dull with no goals to achieve. Negative stress, on the other hand, can lead to physical and mental illness, putting the body in turmoil.

How stress ages the face

Most of us feel severely overstretched trying to balance our work, a family life and social commitments. We feel guilty and become stressed, which instantly ages both our body and face.

Sometimes we overreact and tense up when circumstances don't really warrant it. We become distressed: our faces distort and we find coping with work, illness or personal relationships difficult. Worry (which is wasted energy) manifests itself in clenched jaws, grinding teeth, wild eyes, pallid skin, frowns and involuntary facial movements. You need to recognize the sources of any negative stress in your life (be it a person or event) and then try to avoid them.

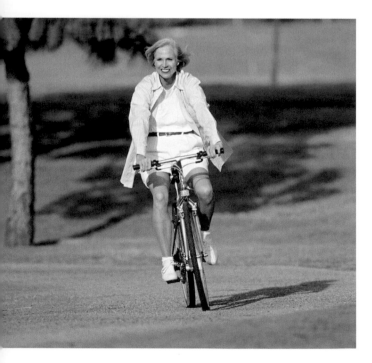

Incorporating exercise into your daily routine is a great way to de-stress and will boost your energy levels.

How stress affects the skin

Stress is a major factor in heart disease, and prolonged stress weakens the immune system, making you more susceptible to minor infections and skin eruptions. Excessive stress creates a bodily state of confusion, strained facial expressions and physical and even mental illnesses.

Stress is instantly visible on the face, and older skins, which possess less elasticity, hang on to stress deep down in the dermis in the form of lines. Stress can send the adrenal glands into overdrive, generate free radicals and decelerate the blood and lymph flow, thereby slowing down the regeneration of skin cells. It can also cause the release of hormones that stimulate the sebaceous glands into overproduction of oil, resulting in break-outs of spots and blemishes.

Sweating causes the skin to become dehydrated and makes it prone to irritation, especially when it combines with make-up. Adult acne may be brought about by stress and its accompanying hormonal fluctuations. Some people rely on props to get them through stressful times, but if your props are chocolate or alcohol, your skin may suffer as a result. Eating a diet high in chocolate and other high-sugar foods can exacerbate pimples, and excessive alcohol consumption can cause tiny veins in the face to dilate and lead to a permanent unsightly network of purple-blue capillaries across the cheeks and nose. Stress overload aggravates eczema or dermatitis, and severe stress can even trigger psoriasis in people who carry the tendency to this condition.

How stress affects the eyes

There are seven important facial muscles concerned with working the eye – but the orbicularis oculi is the major muscle that circles the eye (see pages 50–51). When you overwork and strain your eyes, have difficulties with vision or are in strong sunlight, the orbicularis oculi muscle screws up the eye. Although this screwing up means you can see in more detail, constant overstraining results in lines and wrinkles on your face, as well as painful headaches. Endlessly staring at a computer screen without a break, for example, stresses eye muscles, affects your posture and distorts your face, which, over time, can become permanent. Take a break every 20 minutes or so and treat yourself to the Bright Eyes exercise (see pages 82–83). It will ease tension and banish any headaches.

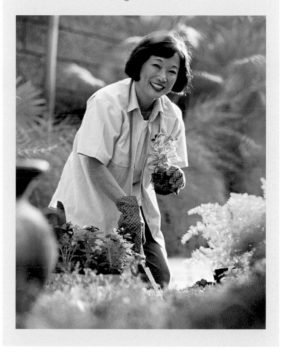

DON'T LET STRESS RUN YOUR LIFE

Take charge of your life and the stress in it. Be physically active: it releases pent-up emotions, stimulates blood and lymph circulation and encourages better sleeping patterns. Whether you like to get hot and sweaty in the gym, take a brisk walk in the park or simply do some gardening – it's completely up to you. It's a good idea, though, to cut down on drinking and stop smoking while you deal with whatever is causing the stress.

Eyes are sensitive not only to bright lights and overwork, but also to excessive dryness. The wind outdoors and the central heating or air conditioning indoors (especially in theatres, cinemas and aircraft) have a drying effect on both the eyes and the skin. Consequently, fewer tears are produced to lubricate the eyes and keep them functioning properly.

Dry eyes feel uncomfortably gritty, but try not to squint and rub them, as this stretches and damages the dry skin around the eyes. This delicate skin then becomes loose and baggy, making your face look old before its time. You can help to combat dehydration, (which can cause dark under-eye circles) and benefit your eyes and skin, by drinking plenty of plain water. This will keep it younger looking and healthier (see pages 112–113).

THINK POSITIVE

Our bodies respond physically to how we feel emotionally. So, having a positive mental approach can work wonders for both your physical health and sense of wellbeing. Have a positive outlook about life in general, and try to think about yourself in positive terms too.

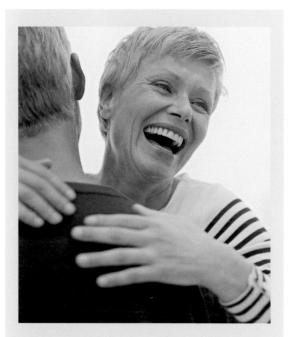

LAUGHING OFF THE LINES

Learn to laugh again. Smiling and laughter release stress-relieving chemicals into the body that lift our mood and help us to relax. Furthermore, the action of laughing lowers blood pressure, exercises the lungs and massages the heart. People who laugh often have good self-esteem and a more positive outlook than those who seldom laugh. A positive attitude to life helps us visibly to delay the ageing process, since expressing positive emotions uses fewer facial muscles than negative emotions. Smiles give out positive signals, helping you and people around you to enjoy life. If you see someone without a smile, give them yours – it could make all the difference and will cost you nothing.

Your face is only a small part of your entire being, but it can tell the world a lot about you. When you look good, you feel good; but you might be surprised to learn just how closely your mind and body track one another. Where one leads, the other is sure to follow, so try to feel good about yourself, and then you will surely look good.

Steady as she goes

Keep yourself on an even keel. Like most things in life, achieving the right balance is key; and this also applies to positive thinking. You need to be able to deal with adversity without becoming depressed, as well as enjoying the highs without going over the top. To relieve stress, a positive attitude is required that allows you time to pay attention to yourself.

Learn to say 'no'

In our busy lives, it can be too tempting to try to do everything that's asked of us. But accepting every party invitation or offering to stay late at work to help a colleague is fine only when it's not a regular demand. Otherwise, you could end up with no time for yourself. Try to prioritize some 'you time' and reorganize other activities around it. Also, try to surround yourself with those people who are true friends and family members and who don't make excessive demands on you.

Get the feel-good factor

Did you know that emotional stress can be eliminated by regular physical activity? So if you exercise on a regular basis, you'll feel happier and have a more relaxed outlook, as well as gaining the physical benefits of better posture, muscle tone and

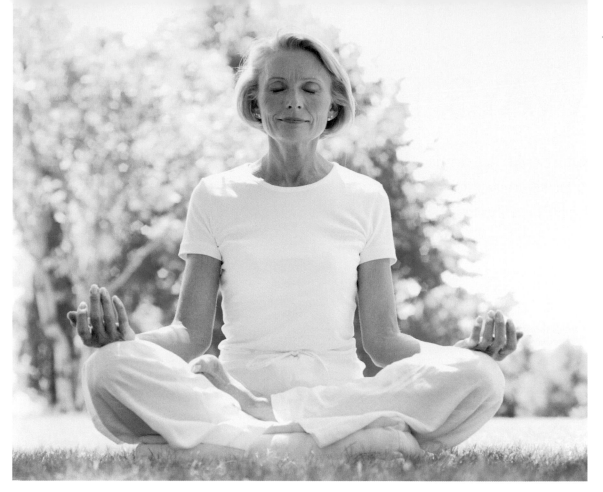

Achieve some inner peace by taking the time to meditate. Just sitting quietly and thinking peaceful thoughts will calm your mind.

circulation. When you exercise, the brain releases chemicals called endorphins, which give you a feel-good factor immediately, and this makes you feel happier about yourself. A more active you will also be healthier and happier and have a glowing complexion.

A mental approach

If swimming, cycling or brisk walking sound too strenuous, consider alternative forms of exercise that have an in-built relaxation element, such as yoga or t'ai chi. Why not try meditation or visualization to influence your mood or give you an instant pick-me-up? Alternatively, just take 10–20 minutes to relax comfortably and quietly with your eyes closed. Focus your mind, discipline yourself to think pleasant thoughts, visualize peaceful places where you are always happy or let a colour that pleases you flood your mind. Sit among plants or perfumes that evoke happy memories, perhaps by burning some joss sticks, and listen to and absorb your favourite music. It is amazing how music and scents can lift your mood, letting you drift away from everyday cares.

BOOST YOUR SELF-CONFIDENCE BY:

- Keeping yourself busy
- Setting yourself achievable goals
- Pursuing your dreams or aspirations
- Furthering your adult education
- Discovering your religious or spiritual side
- Contributing and giving back to society
- Volunteering for charity work
- Keeping in contact with partners, friends and family
- Filling your diary
- Not putting off till tomorrow what can be done today
- Arranging short stays with friends and relatives
- Being sociable, inviting friends and neighbours for drinks – who knows who you might meet?
- Offering to baby-sit for friends or family
- Considering a pet for company (dogs make good walking companions)
- Booking a holiday/residential course to further your hobby
- Pampering yourself

WAYS TO RELAX

After working out your face and body, spend some time relaxing and allowing time for recovery. Breathing is a vital part of relaxation, and you'll need to develop an awareness of your breathing in order to maximize your relaxation potential.

Take a deep breath and relax! The body needs a time of deep relaxation to disperse severe stress, to bring the physical and emotional symptoms of stress under control and replace it with tranquillity.

Try the simple relaxation technique known as The Corpse (see opposite). It may take several attempts for you to relax enough to lie in one position for 20 minutes, but when you are ready, be prepared to sink into pure oblivion while your body is completely limp. When you have finished, open your eyes and slowly return your thoughts to everyday. Get up safely by carefully turning on to your side, then bend your knees and push with your elbows to raise yourself to a kneeling position. Place one foot on the floor, carefully push and stand, slowly uncurling your back, until you are completely upright. Now, stretch both arms above your head, breathe deeply and feel revitalized.

RELAXATION BENEFITS

Mental and physical relaxation help to:
- Release muscular tension
- Release skeletal tension
- Release mental anxiety
- Revive relationships
- Increase a sense of tranquillity
- Boost creativity
- Improve attitude
- Enhance memory
- Lessen pain

Treat yourself

You could relax and pamper yourself with a face, foot or body massage, reflexology, aromatherapy or thalassotherapy (water treatment). These treatments will return your mind and body to a state of calm, reduce your blood pressure and allow you to function more efficiently. Plus, they will boost your circulation of blood and lymph, enabling your body to get on with the job of constant cell renewal, which in turn improves the appearance of your skin.

Where to relax

Achieving a relaxed state of body and mind takes time, so creating a peaceful ambience in which to relax gives you more chance of success. You should be warm, comfortable and free from disturbances.

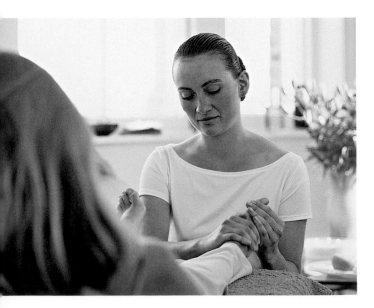

Treat yourself to a reflexology treatment. It will ease your body's aches and pains and put your mind in a serene state.

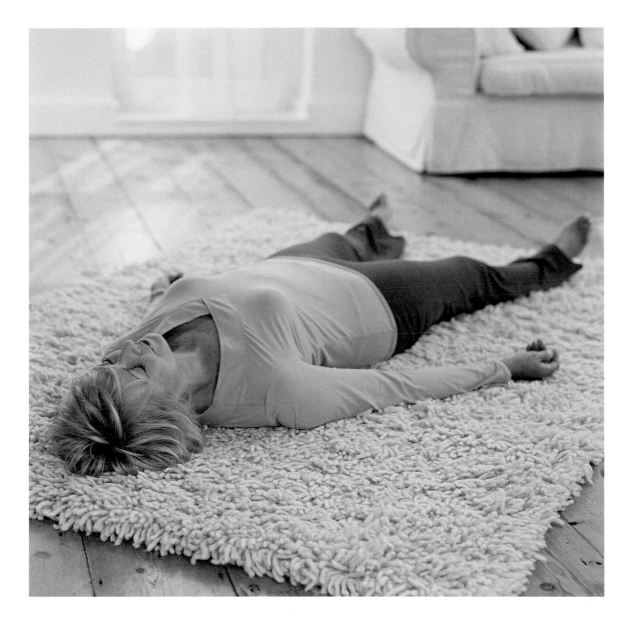

THE CORPSE

1 Lie on your back, with your legs slightly apart and your feet relaxed. Have a blanket nearby in case you feel sleepy afterwards. Take your arms out, slightly away from your body, with your palms facing upwards. Relax your feet and close your eyes. Breathe in through the nose and out through the mouth, with slow, deep breaths. Fill your lungs and concentrate on exhaling slowly; empty your lungs completely before inhaling again. Continue for 2–3 minutes.

2 Tense your toes, feet and knees in turn, then relax them. Then work up through your legs, hips and torso, tensing and relaxing. Now be aware of your fingers, hands and arms, and consciously tense and relax them. Keep moving up your body. You'll need to roll or rotate your shoulders and neck slightly, then screw up and relax your face. Feel your body getting heavier and sinking into the floor. Visualize your place of calm or your favourite colour, and drift away on images and sounds. Breathe normally throughout 20 minutes of tranquillity.

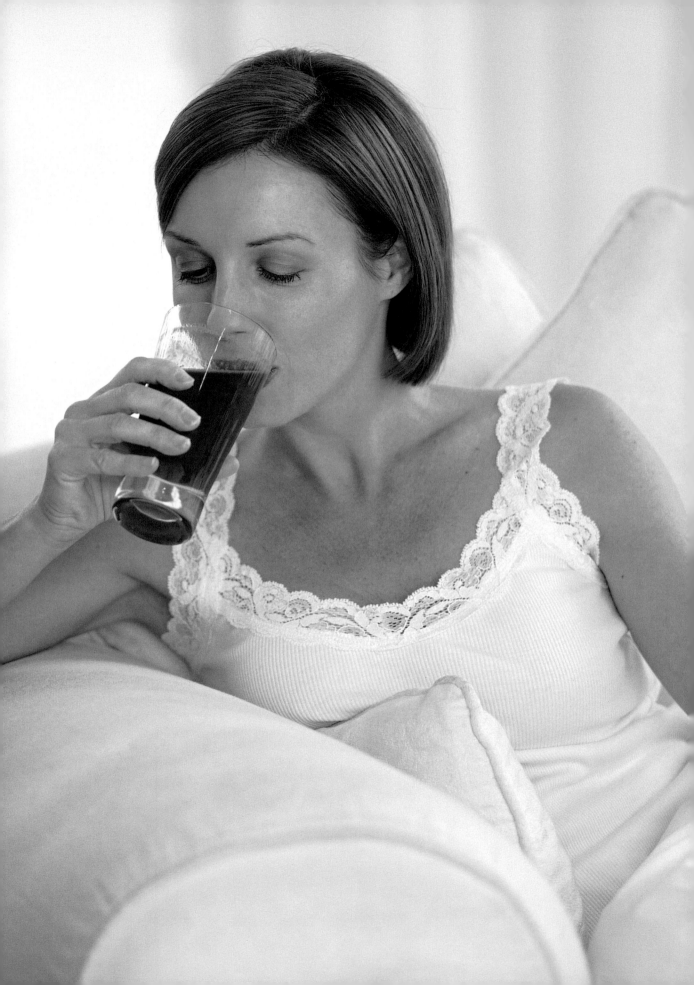

Youth boosters

Destructive free radicals can damage cell membranes, DNA and proteins, causing your skin to age prematurely. But your body can help to counter this potential danger with antioxidants found in youth-boosting foods. You need to learn how to limit your exposure to toxins and restrict the amount entering your body; then the next step is to discover foods that ensure the fast and efficient removal of toxins. Finally, you should find ways to strengthen your detox system, boost your defence mechanisms and create a healthy digestive system.

COMBAT SIGNS OF AGEING

You can help to keep your skin looking great in many simple ways: avoid harmful toxins whenever possible; make body brushing a part of your regular routine; look out for products enriched with natural ingredients and indulge in detoxing baths.

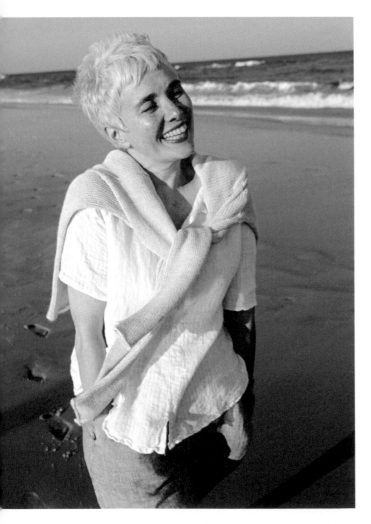

Spending time outside in the fresh air can provide your skin with a welcome break from the de-hydrating effects of air conditioning and central healting.

The next best thing?

Many of the natural ingredients present in today's skin-care and beauty products have been tried and tested over the years. But manufacturers' extensive (and expensive) modern research continuously results in newly discovered ingredients that claim to benefit your skin and are rapidly incorporated into new over-the-counter skin-care products. Keep up to date with products as they appear on the market, but always read the list of ingredients before you buy so you know what the manufacturers are promising. For example, new products containing beta-hydroxy acids (BHAs) claim to assist the skin's natural cell

POLLUTANTS TO AVOID

Read product labels and avoid all of these pollutants:
- Sodium lauryl sulphate
- Sodium laureth sulphate
- Talc
- Mineral oil
- Lanolin
- Tallow
- Aluminium
- Fluorocarbons
- Formaldehyde
- Propylene glycol
- Phthalate

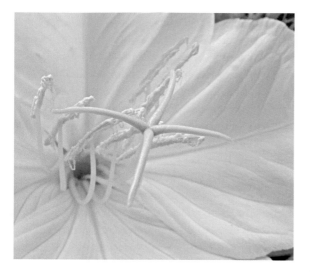

Soothing evening primrose oil is found in many facial moisturizers and hand creams.

A pollutant-free life?

We are exposed to air pollution and other toxins every day of our lives. Pollutants are harmful to the body and are hard to avoid. Many create high levels of free radicals when they enter our system; others act directly on the body's cells to create mutations that could become cancerous. In order to reduce your exposure to pollutants, you need to read product labels on food and household products such as sprays and polishes, toothpaste, mouthwash, antiperspirants and soap, to find out what substances they contain.

Some brands of make-up, skin-care and beauty products may also contain pollutants – and even some baby products need to be scrutinized for potentially harmful substances. Pollutants include pesticides, additives and heavy metals in food and water, gases emitted by photocopiers and printers, and chemicals in cleaning products. (Chemical sensitivity causes common symptoms such as tiredness, rashes and aches and pains that we all too often blame on other causes.) Invisible pollutants can be found in seemingly harmless household goods such as carpets and furnishings as well as electrical equipment.

renewal process and delay outward signs of ageing, whereas products containing panthenol (pro-vitamin B5) claim to improve the skin's condition and encourage the regeneration of skin cells. Look out for skin-care products containing ceramides, which are water-binding agents that help to retain water and keep skin firm and smooth.

Not all products will contain ingredients suitable for your skin, so check that what you want is pH balanced, especially if you have sensitive skin. When you're looking to buy, it's worth considering products found in your local health food shop as well as those on beauty counters in bigger stores.

One of the latest wonder ingredients is DMAE (or dimethylaminoethanol in full), which claims to boost the skin's tone and prevent skin from ageing. At present it's available only through cosmetic surgeons and dermatologists, but keep an eye out for its arrival on beauty counters some time soon.

Look out too for products containing herbal extracts and antioxidants that will benefit your skin naturally and help to keep you looking younger. Aloe vera, an extract of the cactus plant, has been used on the skin since Egyptian times and is known to promote and restore healthy skin. Evening primrose oil is another natural ingredient used in many beauty products. It contains gamma-linolenic acid (usually shortened to GLA) – an essential omega-6 fatty acid that reduces water loss and improves the skin's condition. GLA is also in borage and blackcurrants.

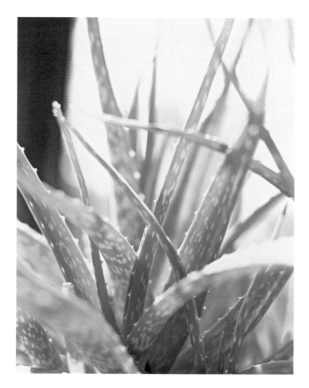

Aloe vera's anti-inflammatory properties are used to treat skin conditions such as psoriasis and burns.

WATER MAKES ALL THE DIFFERENCE

The basic differences between a fresh plum and a shrivelled prune are simply age and water content. If you lie in the sun too much in your youth, you may well be a wrinkly oldie later on, but drinking plenty of water may just tip the balance in your favour.

Your body is composed of two-thirds water and loses at least 1.5 litres (2½ pints) a day; you'll need to drink at least 2 litres (3½ pints) a day for a healthy body and radiant skin. Dehydration causes internal body problems that may well remain invisible, but on the skin's surface problems present as lines and blemishes. It's not on the surface that water is required, it's deep down in the dermis, where your skin cells are 80 per cent liquid and need water to

plump them up. Some people worry that increasing their fluid intake will have them running to the toilet, but bladder capacity naturally increases with water intake.

Get on the wagon

Heavy drinking causes broken blood vessels on the face, dry patches and a pallid, uneven complexion. Too much alcohol the night before also results in 'morning after' headaches, nausea and stomach upsets, and dehydrates internal organs and facial skin. Alcohol robs your body of oxygen and vitamin C and makes blood cells stick together and clog up capillaries, which may rupture, forming thread veins.

Keep your alcohol intake to a minimum. A glass or two of wine a day has been deemed beneficial to health, but, as with many of life's fun things, an excess (more than three glasses a day) is detrimental and speeds up the ageing process.

Many people are permanently dehydrated and suffer from lethargy and headaches simply because they don't drink enough water. As well as keeping you hydrated, water flushes the toxins out of your system. Aim to drink six to eight glasses of clean, filtered water a day, and drink often, sipping from glasses rather than downing one glass at a time. Your urine will be a light straw colour if you drink enough fluid; darker urine indicates dehydration and could possibly lead to the formation of kidney stones.

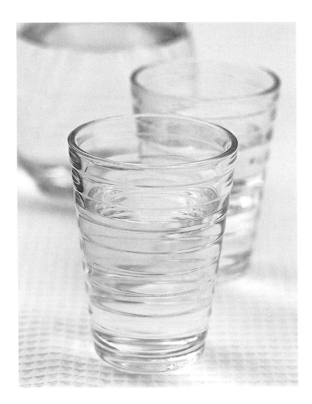

Drinking six to eight glasses of water a day will keep you hydrated and flush out toxins.

Water alternatives

If you're not a great fan of plain water, it's good to know that there are plenty of other drinks to top up your water quota. Milk, for example, is 84 per cent water and herbal infusions and decaffeinated colas are 99 per cent water. Green tea, also rich in antioxidants, makes an ideal drink (and when applied direct to the skin can activate collagen production). Freshly squeezed fruit or vegetable juices are about 90 per cent water, and you get health-giving vitamins thrown in for free.

Boost your water intake by eating water-rich foods such as watermelon, cucumber, celery, grapes and pears. All will increase your fluid intake, but watch their calorie content. Keep off caffeinated drinks because caffeine is a diuretic and so promotes urine loss and you can easily end up dehydrated. Daily food and fluid intake makes all the difference to your digestion and constitution, and constipation or diarrhoea may result if you get it wrong.

A sweaty issue

Nervousness, anger, or hot humid weather conditions can make you 'glow' (a ladylike expression for sweating). It's the body's natural mechanism to make you cool down. Sweating occurs all over the body, including the face (particularly at the time of the menopause), and can be excessive under the arms and, for many people, constant through their feet. In hot climates or when exercising, you need to drink more to replace lost fluids and prevent dehydration.

SPRAY-ON YOUTH

Your body enjoys both internal and external watering. Flat cells on the epidermis are 20 per cent water. Keep them at absorption capacity by splashing your skin often with water. Then, simply pat dry and apply moisturizer immediately to prevent evaporation. Splashing also stimulates your circulation, promotes oil production from sebaceous glands and makes muscles more powerful (the splashing causes them to expand and contract in response). Connective tissues become more flexible, softening expressions.

Carry a small aerosol water spray, or fill your own small spray bottle with distilled or spring water, to refresh tight skin; such a spritz is particularly valuable when flying or in hot weather.

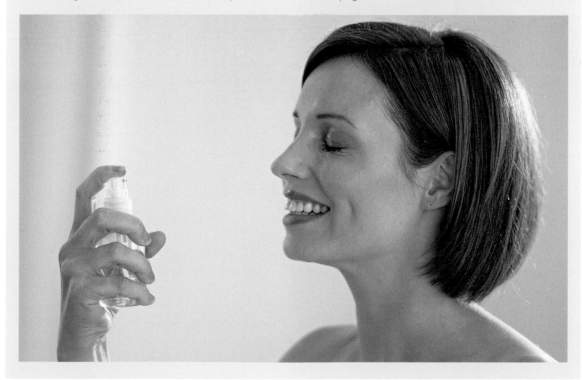

MIRACLE JUICES

The antioxidants present in fruit and vegetables help to combat the free-radical damage that contributes to wrinkles, sagging skin, loss of muscle tone, age spots and the onset of age-related diseases. So the juices below are not only delicious – they're good for you, too.

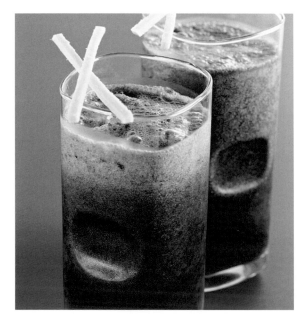

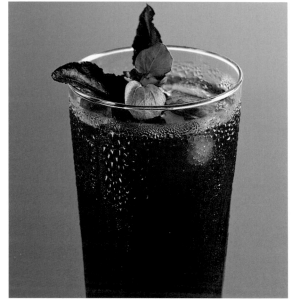

PACKS A PUNCH

Grapefruit is a rich source of vitamin C and bioflavonoids, and blueberries are extremely potent antioxidants.

250 g (8 oz) blueberries
125 g (4 oz) grapefruit
250 g (8 oz) apple
2.5 cm (1 in) cube fresh root ginger, roughly chopped

Juice all the ingredients and serve in a tall glass with ice cubes. Decorate with thin slices of ginger, if liked. Makes 200 ml (7 fl oz).

NUTRITIONAL VALUES

vitamin A 695 iu	niacin 1.91 mg
vitamin C 134 mg	vitamin B6 0.39 mg
magnesium 59 mg	vitamin E 3.12 mg
380 calories	

HEART BEET

Watercress is rich in iron, vitamin C and betacarotene, and onions are good antioxidants.

125 g (4 oz) beetroot
125 g (4 oz) watercress
125 g (4 oz) red onion
250 g (8 oz) carrot
1 garlic clove

Juice the ingredients and serve in a tall glass. Decorate with beet leaves and watercress, if liked. Makes 200 ml (7 fl oz).

NUTRITIONAL VALUES

vitamin A 41,166 iu	niacin 2 mg
vitamin C 85 mg	vitamin B6 0.56 mg
magnesium 85 mg	vitamin E 2.36 mg
167 calories	

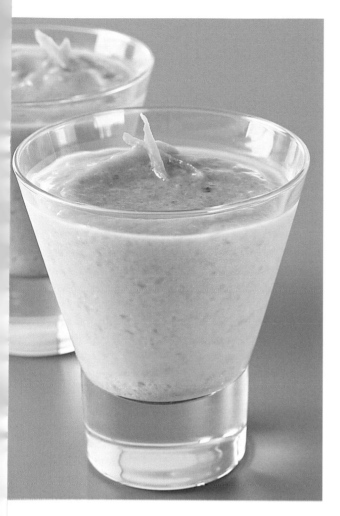

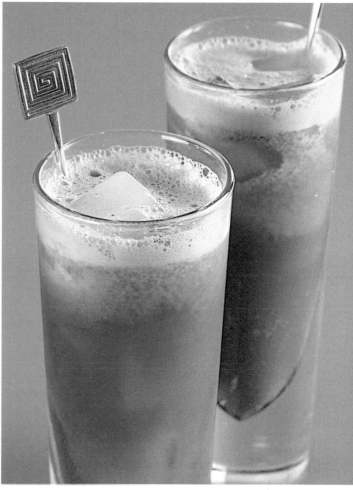

GREEN GODDESS

Avocado is rich in vitamin E and apricots are an excellent source of zinc.

175 g (6 oz) melon (½ large melon)
125 g (4 oz) cucumber
125 g (4 oz) avocado
50 g (2 oz) dried apricots
1 tablespoon wheatgerm

Juice the melon and cucumber. Whizz in a blender with the avocado, apricots, wheatgerm and a couple of ice cubes. Decorate with dried apricot slivers, if liked. Makes 200 ml (7 fl oz).

NUTRITIONAL VALUES

vitamin A 8,738 iu	potassium 1,470 mg
vitamin C 110 mg	iron 1.6 mg
vitamin E 2 mcg	zinc 1.29 mg
357 calories	

SUMMERTIME SIZZLER

All the ingredients in this juice contain high levels of zinc.

125 g (4 oz) asparagus spears
10 dandelion leaves
125 g (4 oz) melon
175 g (6 oz) cucumber
200 g (7 oz) pear

Trim the woody bits off the asparagus spears. Roll the dandelion leaves into a ball and juice them (if you have picked wild leaves, wash them first) with the asparagus. Peel and juice the melon. Juice the cucumber and pear with their skins. Whizz everything in a blender and serve in a tall glass with ice cubes. Makes 200 ml (7 fl oz).

NUTRITIONAL VALUES

vitamin A 5,018 iu	potassium 1,235 mg
vitamin C 87 mg	zinc 1.36 mg
215 calories	

TOP 20 DETOX FOODS

These top 20 detox foods have been shown to provide the best all-round nutrients that will work hard to get rid of the toxins in your body.

1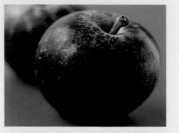

APPLES are an excellent source of vitamin C and quercetin – an antioxidant that lowers fat and cholesterol levels. They also contain pectin – a soluble fibre that binds heavy metals (such as mercury and lead) in the colon, encouraging their removal from the body.

2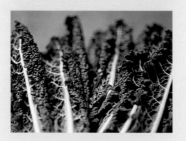

GARLIC boosts the immune system. When crushed, it releases the chemical allicin, which converts to a sulphur-based compound in the body that combines with harmful chemicals, food additives and metal toxins to be excreted as one package. Sulphur fights nicotine addiction, reducing toxin levels.

3

CRUCIFEROUS VEGETABLES, including cauliflower, cabbage, spinach, kale and Brussels sprouts, are extremely powerful detoxers. They contain glucosinolates, which prompt the liver to produce vital enzymes that neutralize particular toxins.

4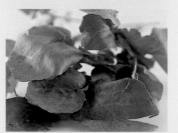

WATERCRESS contains the green pigment of plants – chlorophyll. This iron-rich pigment helps to build red blood cells and boosts the body's circulation. It increases the detox enzymes and helps to eliminate carcinogens caused by smoking.

5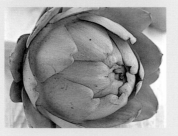

ARTICHOKES contain antioxidant chemicals and increase bile production. Bile carries harmful toxins, which are not water soluble, to the bowel or kidneys for excretion, and artichoke increases its rate of flow.

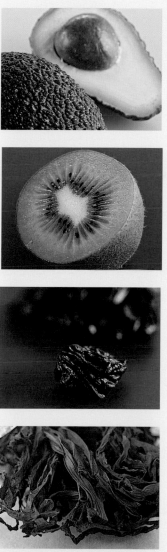

AVOCADOS contain essential fatty acids and glutathione – an age-protective antioxidant that fights free radicals. Glutathione combines with fat-soluble toxins such as alcohol, making them available for excretion.

KIWI FRUIT is a powerful antioxidant packed with vitamin C that helps the body to manufacture the detoxer glutathione. (Levels of glutathione can increase by 50 per cent in two weeks.)

PRUNES are a fantastic antioxidant food, with blueberries coming a close second. As you may expect, prunes contain a natural laxative – tartaric acid – and dihydrophenylisatin, a substance that stimulates the intestines. By making the bowel work efficiently, they eliminate waste and reduce toxic reabsorption.

SEAWEED contains high levels of the minerals magnesium, calcium, iron and iodine. These seaweed alginates bind to radioactive material and heavy metals for the body to eliminate as waste.

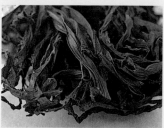

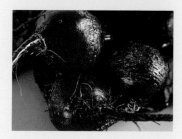

BEETROOT contains the essential amino acid methionine, which helps to purify body waste products and reduce cholesterol levels. It has been used since Roman times for blood purifying, and contains ingredients that may absorb toxic metals. Other micronutrients within beetroot are folate, potassium and manganese, and its tops are packed with calcium, betacarotene and iron.

DETOX FOR PERFECT SKIN

Toxins are harmful substances detrimental to health that are found in products, foods and the environment. We constantly overload our bodies with them, but how can we avoid them?

If your body suffers from toxic build-up, you should detox and clean your system. Modern life and fast lifestyles can be the major contributors to toxin overload, causing tiredness or even exhaustion. Your body becomes overwhelmed, and you need to remove toxins to function efficiently again. Your body has a natural toxin elimination system, but constant exposure to toxins makes it difficult to keep your body toxin-free. Your body's detox system consists of:

- Liver
- Kidneys
- Fat stores
- Lungs
- Lymphatic system
- Bowel
- Skin

This natural detox system should, in theory, keep you clear from toxic troubles – provided all seven components are kept in good working order. But if just one component fails, toxins that are not eradicated will build up. A hangover is a good example of this. When you drink too much, your liver cannot process the excess alcohol at the same rate as it is being drunk. Consequently, excess toxins begin to pile up and poison your body, causing nausea, headache and an upset stomach. As time passes, the liver copes with elimination and the unpleasant symptoms subside.

Smoking is another example of pushing your detox system past its capabilities. Your lungs contain low levels of antioxidants, which neutralize free radicals and convert toxins into water-soluble substances that we exhale. Smoking stresses the lungs with excessive

toxins, which build up and stress your detox system. It also causes internal poisoning, creating problems of less energy, poor immunity from disease, weight gain, cellulite and even arthritis.

The aim of the detox plan

Detoxing is a focused effort to:

- Clear blood and lymph system of toxic rubbish
- Reduce toxic build-up
- Boost defence mechanisms
- Neutralize harmful toxins
- Reduce toxin damage
- Boost blood flow
- Strengthen the power of skin and lungs
- Increase levels of natural enzymes in the liver

This detox plan is not a diet to lose weight and you don't have to starve yourself – far from it. You could apply the detox plan for just a week, but it is better still to make it a permanent part of your lifestyle. You could also start by introducing some of the aspects of the plan, then gradually include other aspects later, rather than making a dramatic change in your diet and lifestyle all at once.

The main aim of detoxing is to work with your body and limit the amount of toxins entering it. This is not an easy task, but reducing the amount of toxins your body is exposed to reduces the pressure on your natural detox system. You can strengthen your existing detox system by increasing your consumption of foods that boost the levels of natural enzymes produced in your body. For example, natural enzymes in your liver transform toxins into a water-soluble form for

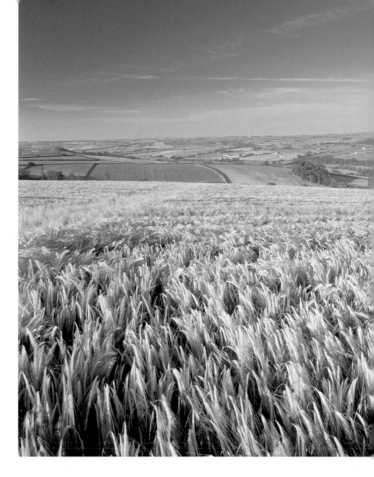

Escape to the country for an invigorating break from the toxins encountered in city life.

excretion, so eating foods that stimulate your bowel to work efficiently will clear your blood and lymph systems of toxic rubbish.

How to follow the plan

Conscientiously eat good, nutritious food, drink plenty of water and balance your food intake with regular exercise and a positive attitude – it's that simple.

- Reduce your calories: aim for a low-calorie, high-nutrient diet (i.e. one based primarily on fruit and vegetables and wholegrain carbohydrates). Cutting your calories to around 1,500 a day if you are a woman, or 2,000 a day if you are a man, is ideal.
- Eat less fat: no more than 30 per cent of your daily calories should come from fat, with less than 10 per cent of these coming from saturated fats, such as fatty meat and hard cheese.
- Eat less sugar: eating less than 40 g (1½ oz) a day will cut down on the number of free radicals in your body and also decrease your chance of developing Type II diabetes, which can take 20 years off your life.
- Aim to eat at least five servings a day of the detoxing fruit and vegetables on pages 118–121.
- Eat garlic: eat fresh garlic every day, and also take supplements to keep your heart working well.
- Exercise regularly: exercise lowers blood pressure, strengthens the heart, decreases body fat and lowers stress levels. It also makes you feel great!
- Think positively: negative emotions depress our immune system, making us more prone to illness. So having a positive attitude also keeps your body healthy.
- Keep an alert mind: the saying 'use it or lose it' is highly applicable to the brain. If you keep your brain active, you will keep it healthy for longer.

Avoid 'quick-fix' detox diets

So-called 'detox diets' rarely work as they are too low in calories and, being devoid of carbohydrates, cause the body's metabolic rate to grind to a halt. Within two days of starting such a diet, all body processes will have slowed down, including those involved with waste removal, due to the lack of fibre intake. Slowing down the rate of waste elimination results in a sluggish bowel, which is unable to rid the body efficiently of toxins included in body waste.

DETOX BASICS

- Cut down on alcohol. Up to two glasses a day is beneficial, but anything more than that, particularly binge drinking, can attack major organs, brain cells and vision.
- Stop smoking. Cigarettes contain the stimulant nicotine, which is highly addictive. When tobacco is burnt, thousands of harmful poisons are inhaled, including lead, arsenic and cyanide-containing toxins. In addition, carbon monoxide starves the body of oxygen and smoking promotes the production of chemicals called nitrosamines, which cause cancer.
- Reduce exposure to toxins. Pesticides are toxic. Toxins are found in insecticides, garden produce and insect sprays, and your body finds these especially hard to detox.
- Cut back on caffeinated drinks such as tea, coffee and colas, though note that green tea is a highly beneficial drink. Drink plain water or other water alternatives (see page 113) instead.

QUICK-REFERENCE GUIDE

Use this quick-reference guide as an *aide-mémoire* to remind you of the sequence of facial exercises within the fresh face workout. It should remind you at a glance how to do each exercise, so that you can perform a series of exercises in one session.

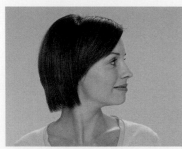

1 Look Out: shoulders facing front; look right; look left.

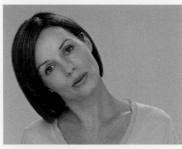

2 Stretch Out: right ear over right shoulder; left ear over left.

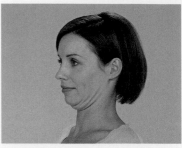

3 Chicken Neck: chin parallel with floor; chin out; pull back.

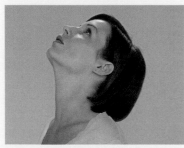

4 The Swan: head back; stretch out neck and hold.

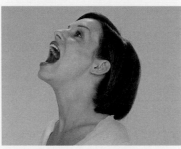

5 The Goldfish: head back; stretch neck; stick out chin – glug.

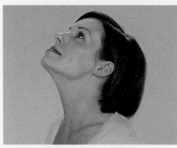

6 The Pelican: head back; stretch neck; push chin and teeth forward – bite.

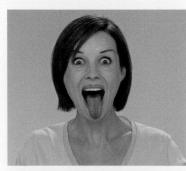

7 The Lion: open eyes wide; fingers out; tongue out – roar.

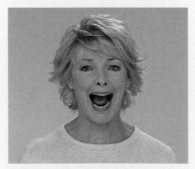

8 Do As I Say: mouth open; say 'uh', 'ee', 'ah'.

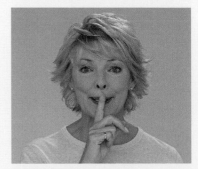

9 Whistlestop: lips taut across teeth; finger middle; whistle.

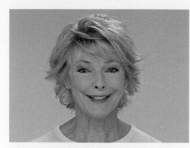

10 The Joker: mouth open; lips narrow; pull up corners – smile.

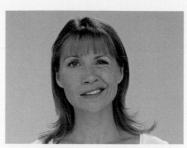

11 The Snarl: lips together; lift; snarl right; snarl left.

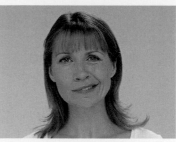

12 The Cheshire Cat: lips together; lift; smile right; smile left.

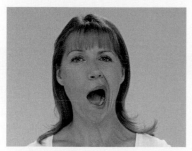

13 The Cow: lift cheeks; lift; chew cud right; chew cud left.

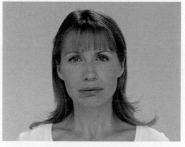

14 Blow Out: lips together; blow out cheeks; slowly blow out mouth.

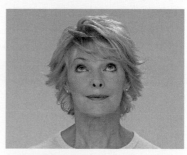

15 Bright Eyes: head still; eyes right, down; left, up.

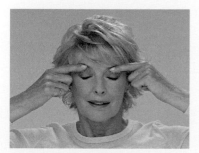

16 Uppers: forefingers above eye sockets; blink rapidly.

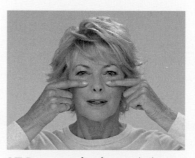

17 Downers: forefingers below eyes; squeeze up lower lids; small movement.

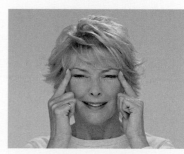

18 Crow's Feet: forefingers corner of eyes; squint and resist.

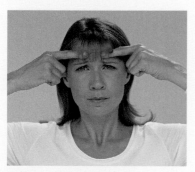

19 Cross Lines: forefingers inner corner eyebrows; frown together.

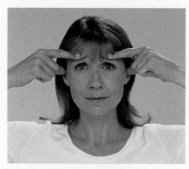

20 Life Lines: forefingers above eyebrows; close eyes; open wide.

INDEX

ACKNOWLEDGEMENTS

Author acknowledgements

For my 'sisters' throughout the world to inform and encourage.

With special thanks to my family and close friends for their continuing love and encouragement. And to Martyn 'the make-up' Fletcher for his professional help and support regarding all aspects of beauty and make-up.

Grateful thanks to Sarah Tomley and Alison Goff at Hamlyn, and also Tony Fitzpatrick at TFA Group, who all believed in me and made this project happen.

Picture acknowledgements

Special Photography: © Octopus Publishing Group Limited/Mike Prior

Other Photography:Alamy/Plantography 109 top
Corbis UK Ltd/Philip Harvey 22/Jutta Klee 102/ROB & SAS 108
Creatas/Imagesource 13 bottom left, 13 top right
Getty Images 15/Peter Adams 123/Ron Chapple 101/Chris Craymer 111 bottom /Emmanuel Faure 13 top left/Frederic Lucano 103/Mark Scott 100/Paul Viant 111 top /Paul Vozdic 13 bottom right/Simon Watson 109 bottom
Imagestate/Pierre Bourrier 23
Octopus Publishing Group Limited/Frank Adam 120 centre left top/Jean Cazals 117/Stephen Conroy 114 left, 114 right, 115 left, 115 right, 118 centre left top, 119 top left, 119 centre left, 119 bottom left, 119 centre left top, 121 centre left bottom/Jeremy Hopley 118 centre left bottom/David Jordan 118 top left/Sandra Lane 118 centre left/Gary Latham 116, 121 bottom left/William Lingwood 121 centre left top/David Loftus 121 centre left/Lis Parsons 121 top left/William Reavell 1, 21, 51, 120 top left, 120 centre left, 120 bottom left/Craig Robertson 120 centre left bottom/Gareth Sambidge 20/Ian Wallace 104, 118 bottom left, 119 centre left bottom

Publisher acknowledgements

Executive Editor Sarah Tomley
Editor Charlotte Wilson
Executive Art Editor Karen Sawyer
Designer Peter Gerrish
Senior Production Controller Martin Croshaw
Picture Researcher Jennifer Veall
Photographer Mike Prior
Hair and Makeup Martyn Fletcher
Models Sally Way, Frances Wingate
Illustration Kevin Jones Associates

Hamlyn would very much like to thank the following for suppling products for photography:

Clarins for the supply of beauty products
Clarins (UK) Ltd, Cavendish Place, London W1M 0DN
00 44 (0)20 7307 6700
www.clarins.com

Hards PR Limited for the supply of Marks and Spencer beauty products
The Hall, Peyton Place, Greenwich, London SE10 8RS
00 44 (0)20 8293 7150
www.hardspr.com

L'Oreal for the supply of beauty products
L'Oreal (UK) Ltd, 255 Hammersmith Road, London W6 8 AZ
00 44 (0)20 8762 4000
www.loreal.com

Marks and Spencer for the loan of clothing from their View From sportswear range and for the supply of beauty products
458 Oxford Street, London W1C 1AP
00 44 (0)20 7935 7954
www.marksandspencer.com